SEAFOOD RECIPES

from the

ADRIATIC SEA

in

ITALY

GIANNI SCASSA

Paperback: 978-1-961438-45-3
eBook: 978-1-961438-46-0
Library of Congress Control Number: 2023912550

This Book is a work of non-fiction

Ordering Information:

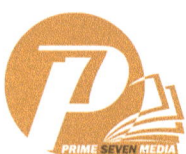

Prime Seven Media
518 Landmann St.
Tomah City, WI 54660

Printed in the United States of America

Professor Ghiottone Fish Recipes from the Adriatic Sea
What I can cook only for Love and Sympathy
The recipes are not to be found on the Internet,
or if there are, they are wrong.

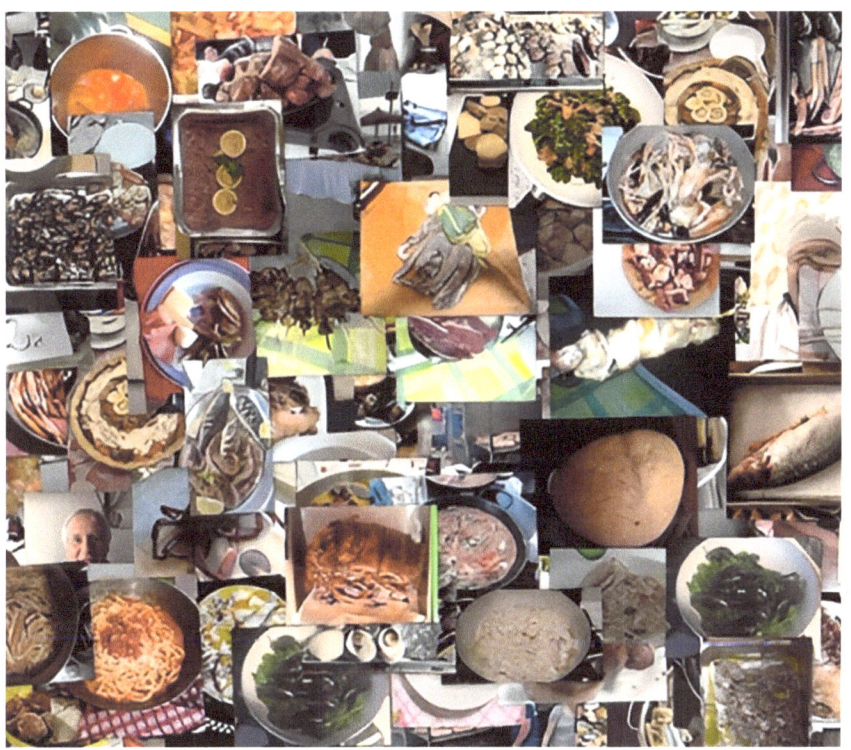

Family recipes revisited by gluttony.

EDITIONS
On my own
Carmina non dant panem
Gianni Scassa

Index

Warning

When you cook these dishes, learn the following special procedures, as explained in the recipes.

1 Cooking pasta the way Risotto is cooked, that is, adding gradually sauce or broth to the pasta, until it is cooked, without boiling it in hot water.

3 Squeezing of the scampi heads in the base for the sauce.

4 Broth with squeezed scampi heads.

5 Toasting in olive oil of the dried red peppers; one per person

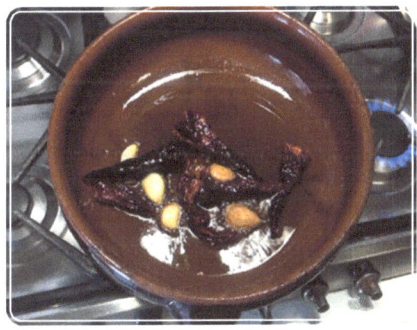 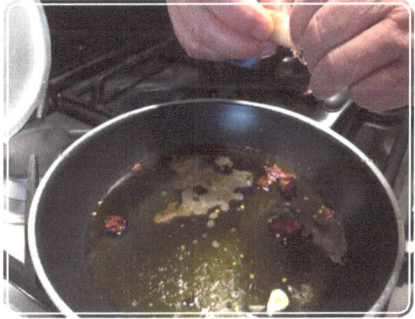

Soon as   5   3

I'll have no other starter but you.

1) Raw Squid from the Adriatic Sea

Yes, just from the Adriatic, because there are defrosted blocks of squid from the most remote seas of the earth.

- ❀ If you don't eat the eyes of the squids, it means that you can't appreciate it.

The Fishermen of Borgo Marino say.

DIRECTIONS

Remove the small transparent cartilage pen from the squid, being careful not to break the bag with the black liquid; if you really don't like it, take its eyes off too.

Put the cleaned baby squid in salted water.
Shake them from time to time, changing the water every half hour and always rising, until it stops producing foam; time needed a couple of hours.

Drain the squid and dry them well with absorbent kitchen paper.

Arrange them in a bowl, put the onion cut into thin slices, the vinegar in moderate quantities, the olive oil and the fresh green chili pepper if in season, or the dry red one.
Serve the raw with toasted bread.

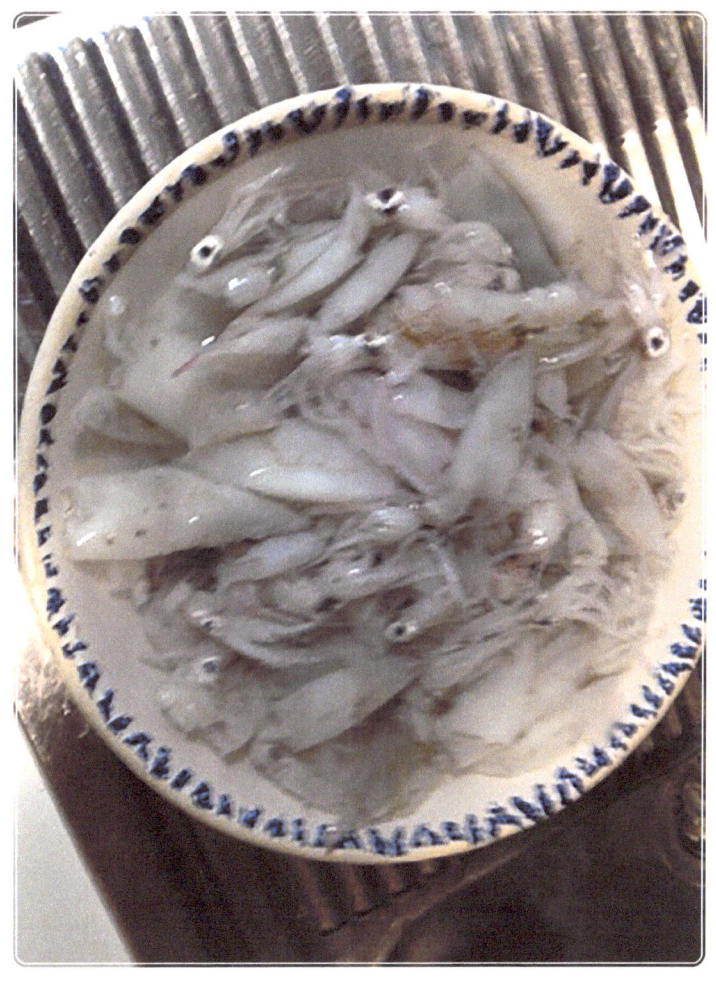

Passion for Mussels

2) Homemade noodles with mussels and Pecorino Cheese from Farindola

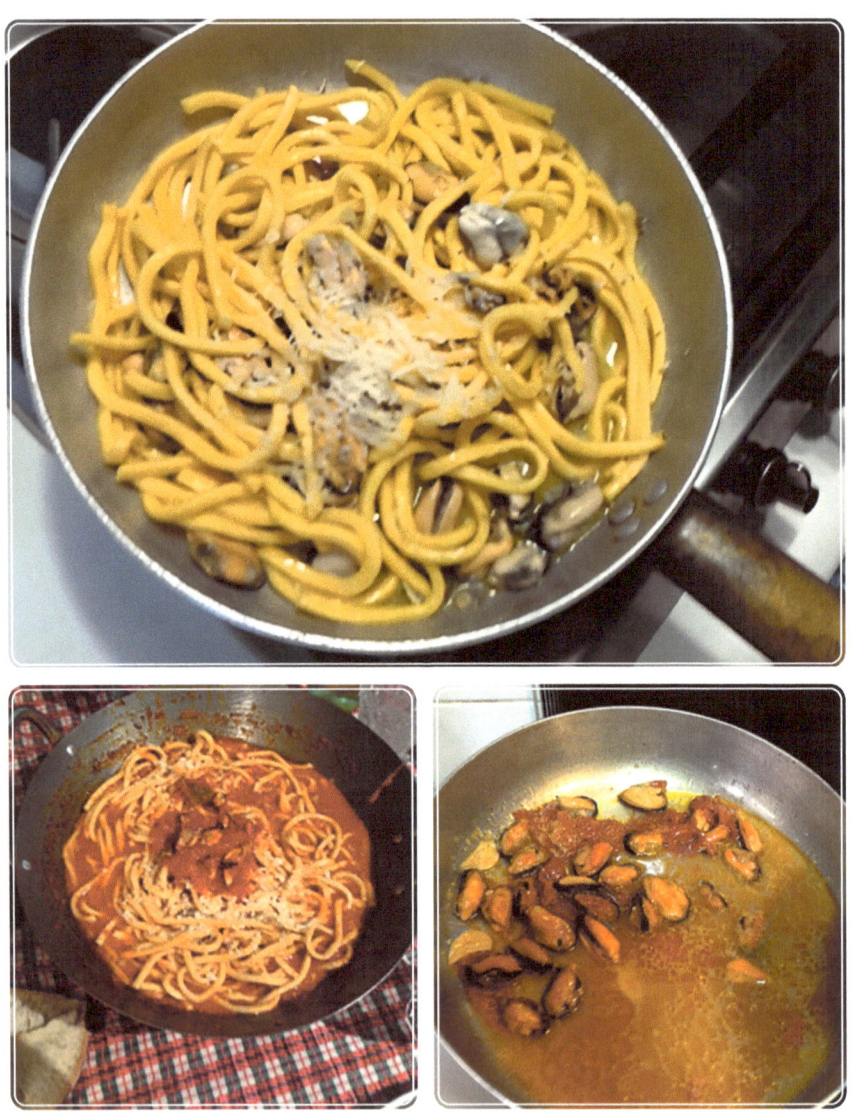

white or with tomato sauce

Homemade egg (*pasta alla chitarra*) in its thicker variety *(chitarrone)* seasoned with fish sauce, or with seafood is the flagship of Abruzzo fish-based cuisine. The mussels match perfectly with Abruzzo pecorino of excellence.

INGREDIENTS and doses for four people, normal eaters.

1. One and a half kg of good quality mussels, at least twelve per person.
2. 1 cherry tomato every three people.
3. 50/70 gr of pecorino di Farindola, or if you prefer pecorino di Fossa.
4. Half a kg of egg pasta alla chitarra.
5. Garlic, oil, parsley, and hot pepper.
6. Fresh green pepper.
7. A sprig of rosemary.

DIRECTIONS

After cleaning the mussels by depriving them of the "mustache" (Byssus), in a pan fry oil, garlic, a sprig of rosemary, a stem of parsley and some pieces of green pepper[*].

When garlic is well browned, add the mussels with half a glass of water and open them over high heat; be careful, as soon as they open turn off the heat, prolonging the cooking they dry, while they must be just burned.

_____

[*] The procedure of opening the fruits in oil, can also be done for spaghetti with clams, or other seafood in white and red (Not for clams of the Adriatic, which express their best in white sauce).

Shell the mussels and set aside with the cooking water.

In a pan prepare a sauce with oil, garlic, and fresh cherry tomatoes, after having blanched them for a minute and deprived of the skin.

In a little filtered water from the mussels, cook the chitarrone for a few minutes. Pay attention to the salt, no salt if you have enough water from the mussels to *Risottare* the pasta alla chitarra, a little if you have added normal water to the mussel water.

Risottare means: to cook the pasta, as if it were a risotto, covering it with a little water at the time and gradually adding the already tasty and hot cooking liquids, such as mussel water, fish broth and fish court bouillon, or meat broths and vegetables.

Add the remaining water to the sauce, the shelled mussels and two or three mussels per person with their shells.

Finish cooking the "pasta alla chitarra" stir-fry it in its sauce.
Grate the pecorino di Farindola or Fossa into thin flakes over the pasta.

For those who love tomatoes, there is a red version of this dish, where the chitarrone is replaced by Pasta alla Mugnaia (Miller) another flagship of Abruzzo cuisine; for the red version the sauce will be more consistent and only when it is cooked the mussels will be added and their water will be amalgamated into the sauce, without diluting the sauce too much.

White version

Linguine with mussels with garlic, olive oil, "fuffulloni", chili and pecorino di Fossa

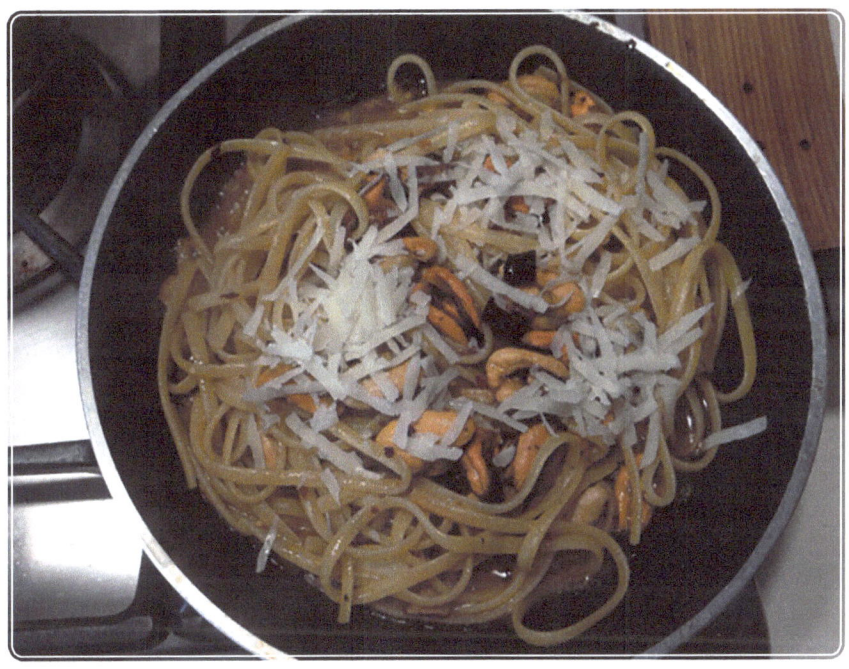

3) Orecchiette (Homemade Pasta) with turnip greens and mussels.

We like Puglia, so let's pay it a tribute.

INGREDIENTS

1. 10/12 mussels of good size.
2. 600 grams of leaves of tender turnip.
3. Garlic, oil, salt, and pepper.
4. half a glass of white wine
5. Two or three anchovy fillets in oil.
6. 80 grams of Apulian orecchiette per person.

DIRECTIONS

Put a little oil in a pan, three or four cloves of dressed garlic, heat the oil and melt the anchovy fillets.

Add the tenderest leaves of the turnips, half a glass of water, half of white wine, coarse salt at your discretion, cover and simmer the turnips over low heat.

When they are cooked al dente and never soft, chop them with a knife and set aside with the cooking liquid.

Without washing it, in the same cooking pan as the turnips, put a veil of oil, peeled garlic at your discretion and when the oil is hot, put the mussels with the shells and let them open.

As the mussels open, even if still half raw, remove them from the heat and remove the shell immediately.

Cook the orecchiette in water with a little salt, drain them al dente and finish cooking in the same pan as the mussels and turnips.

Finally, add the turnip greens leaves cut with a knife with their cooking liquid and the shelled mussels to the orecchiette.

Stir in the orecchiette and check the salting.

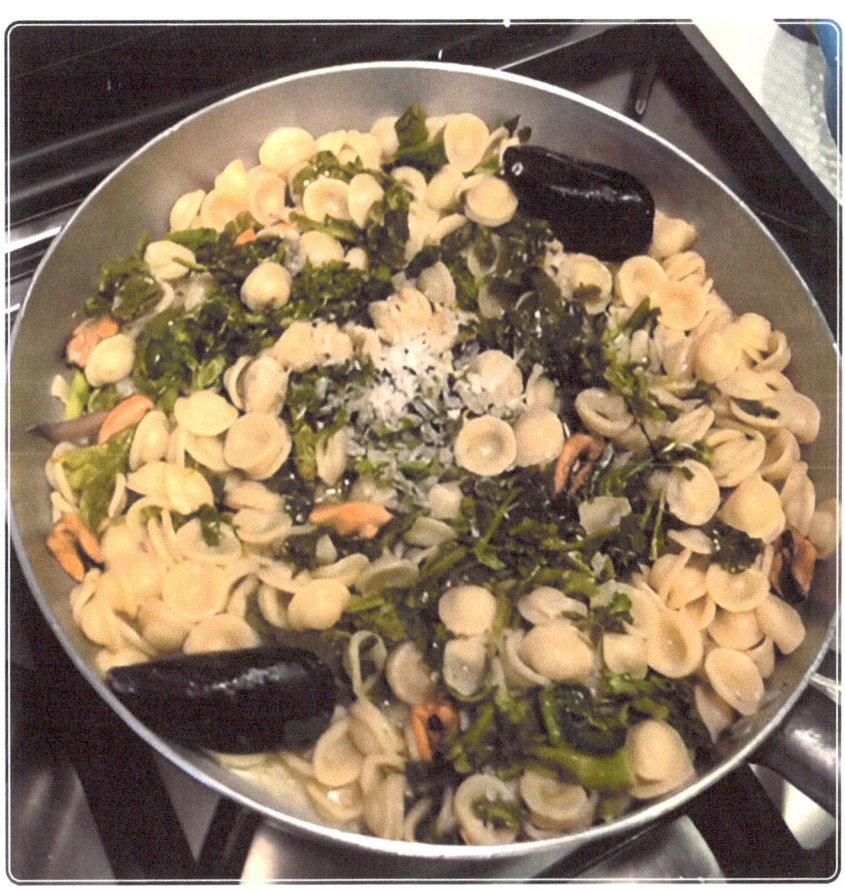

4) Homemade egg pasta with wild mussels from of the Central Adriatic Sea

This type of mussels is rarely found for sale. It can be tasted only if fished from the rocky areas of the central Adriatic coast and the Abruzzo coast of the Trabocchi.

INGREDIENTS

1. One and a half kg of non-farmed mussels, at least 12 per person.
2. 1 cherry tomato every three people.
3. 80 grams of De Cecco spaghetti alla chitarra per person, or other quality pasta of your choice.
4. Garlic, oil, parsley and hot pepper, green if it is in season, or dry red which is always available.
5. Fresh green pepper
6. A sprig of rosemary

DIRECTIONS

Veil the bottom of the pan with good extra virgin olive oil, put the garlic, cherry tomatoes, and mussels well washed and deprived of the "mustache," following the procedure of opening the fruits in oil referred to in recipe 2.

At the same time, start cooking the spaghetti alla chitarra in water with a little salt.

While the mussels open and release the liquid, drain the almost raw spaghetti and finish cooking in the liquid of the mussels and the sauce. Check the salting of the pasta as the liquid of the mussels is already salty.

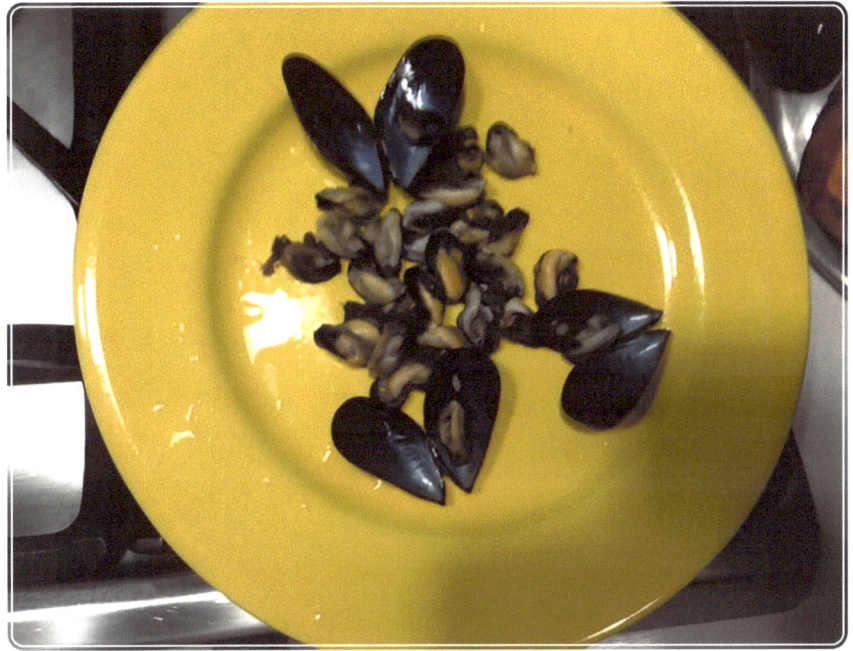

5) Homemade bread with mussels on top

It took fifty years of quarrels and discussions about what was the best way to cook mussels, without pasta: sauté? Peppery? Sauté? Eventually, one day ...

INGREDIENTS

1. 12/20 mussels of good farm quality per person, better if fished from the rocks.
2. olive oil
3. Freshly ground green pepper.
4. Juice of one lemon
5. Mussel water.
6. Home-made bread.

DIRECTIONS

Open the mussels over high heat, removing them as they open.

Carefully filter the cooking water of the mussels.

Open the mussels by removing the shell without stalk, leaving them in the other and arrange them one by one in good order.

In a cup, mix a ladle of mussel water with olive oil, pepper, and lemon juice until you get a thick sauce.

Sprinkle the open mussels with the sauce and keep them in the fridge for five minutes.

Sprinkle slices of good homemade bread with the sauce and more olive oil and enjoy them with the mussels.

A good Brut Sparkling Wine will suit the mussels well.

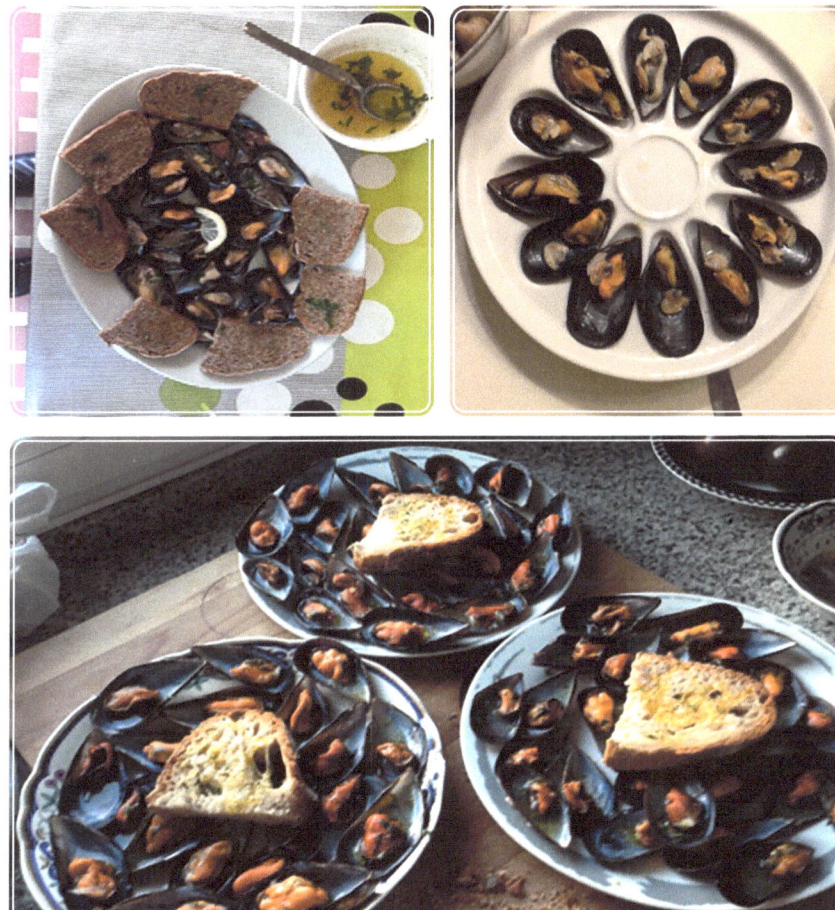

First dishes dancing

6) Spaghetti garlic, extra virgin olive oil, chili pepper and "panocchie" (Squilla).

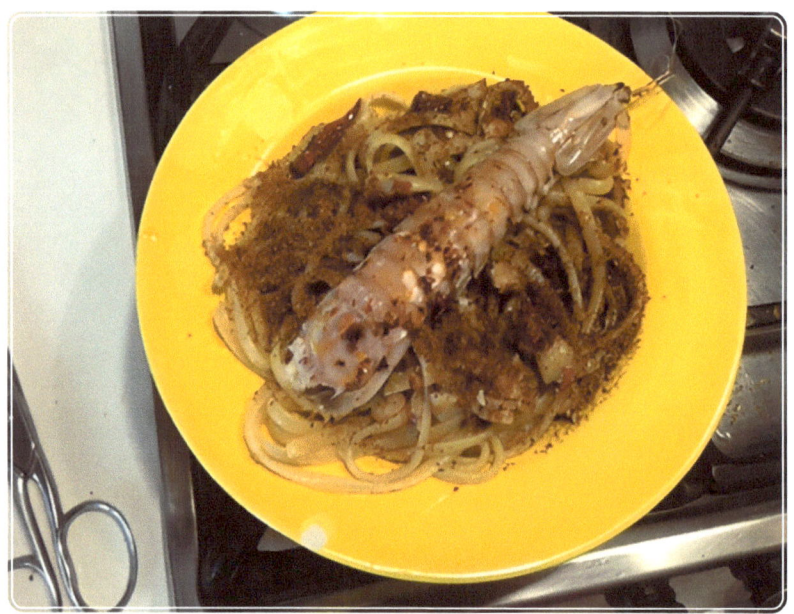

INGREDIENTS

1. 2/3 fresh squillas per person.
2. 3/4 cloves of garlic per person, plus 2/3 cloves for each additional person.
3. A fillet of anchovies in oil.
4. A hot pepper, salt just enough.
5. Quality extra virgin olive oil, just enough to veil the bottom of the pan.
6. Large spaghetti, eighty grams, or more per person.
7. One tablespoon of good quality breadcrumbs per person.

DIRECTIONS

In a pan heat the olive oil and put the garlic cloves cut into small wheels and the chili pepper into small pieces. If the garlic is not appreciated, you can decrease the quantity, but the dish will no longer be Spaghetti with garlic, oil, and chili!

Melt an anchovy fillet in the hot oil, without frying it and squeeze a few heads of the squillas, in the sauce and add a little cooking water from the pasta.

Brown the garlic well and add salt. To prevent them from burning, remove and put the pan back on the heat, then add the squillas cut into pieces and cook for a few minutes.

Cook the spaghetti, drain them al dente and finish cooking by skipping them directly into the base sauce; *any dryness of the pasta and the sauce are corrected by adding water to the pasta.*
Toast the breadcrumbs making it brown and put it on the spaghetti.

Version with shrimp for a friend

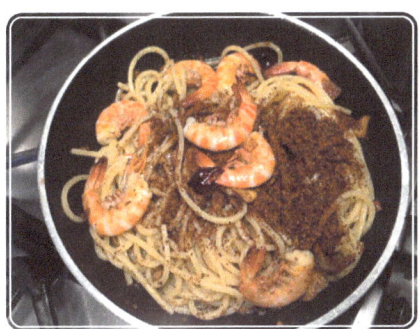 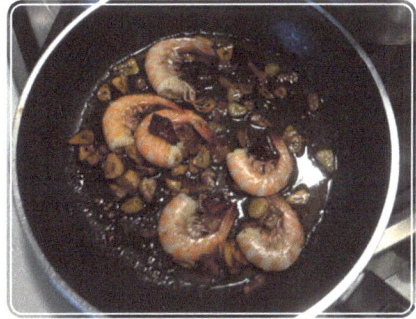

7) Paccheri with scampi

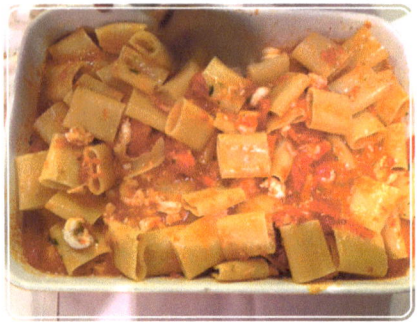 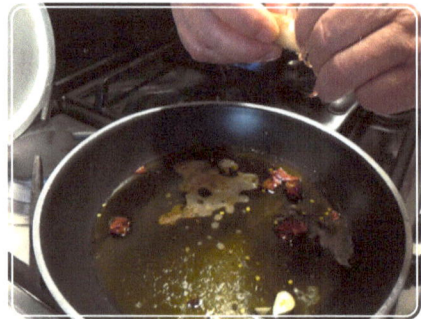

Squeezing of the heads of the scampi

It is one of the most popular dishes in fish restaurants. A super classic offered by everyone, but here is a magic ... Someday I'll tell you!*

INGREDIENTS

1. 2/3 fresh scampi per person (alternatively frozen ones can also be used, provided they are thawed slowly at room temperature and not in water.)
2. 3/4 cherry tomatoes per person.
3. A little good Cognac.
4. Quality paccheri; eighty gr per person.
5. Just enough oil to veil the bottom of the pan.
6. Garlic, a clove.

---

* The magic is squeezing the head of the scampi in the oil.

DIRECTIONS

Remove the head from the scampi and shell the tails.

Peel the scampi (see tutorial on YouTube).

Heat the oil, lightly brown the garlic, and remove it if you don't like it.

Squeeze the heads of the scampi into the oil.

They will release the liquid and the soft parts.

Boil the squeezed scampi heads in a little water, to have a "court bouillon."

Add a little Cognac to the base and let it evaporate quickly by raising the heat.

Add the crushed tomatoes and salt the sauce to taste.

Cook the mixture for twenty minutes, adding a few tablespoons of "court bouillon", if necessary to prevent the sauce from shrinking too much.

Add the shelled scampi tails only in the last five minutes of cooking the sauce and blanch them until they turn pink.

Cook the quality Paccheri, adding the residual "court bouillon" to the water, drain them "al dente" finish cooking in the sauce and add some chopped parsley, if desired.

The "*Risottatura*" of pasta, as explained above, is always to be preferred, in this case use the boiling water of the squeezed prawn heads.

8) Bucatini with sardines and fennel leaves (Modified Sicilian recipe)

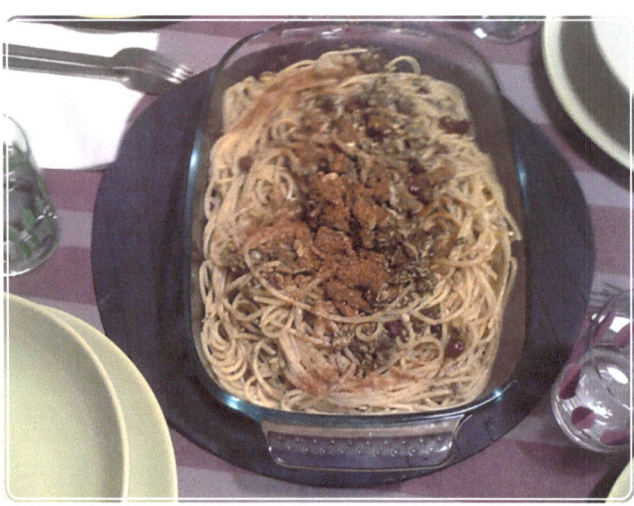

Perhaps the sultana grapes and pine nuts of the original Sicilian recipe do not meet the favor of the Abruzzo's taste. Let's betray Sicily.

INGREDIENTS and doses for 4/6 people; you are, if normal; 4, if a voracious fork.

1. 600 grams of fresh sardines.
2. 4/5 salted anchovies.
3. A large bunch of wild fennels, which if unavailable can be replaced with fennel beard.
4. 2/3 tablespoons of double tomato concentrate.
5. Half an onion and a clove of garlic.
6. 20 gr of raisins, in the original Sicilian recipe, but can be eliminated if the sweetish taste is not appreciated.
7. A handful of pine nuts.
8. A handful of ground almonds.

9. One tablespoon per person of good quality breadcrumbs
10. Extra virgin olive oil, just enough to veil the bottom of the pan.
11. 600 grams of not too big bucatini, or short pasta.
12. a spoonful coffee of saffron.

DIRECTIONS

In a saucepan with high sides of sauce, in the veil of extra virgin oil, which caresses the bottom, gently fry the finely chopped onion and a clove of garlic, if desired.

While the garlic and onion are browning, add the salted anchovies, desalted in water, and deprived of the bone, which will soon liquefy in the hot oil and amalgamate with the onion will form the bottom of the sauce.

Meanwhile, boil the fennel in lightly salted water, which must be softened during cooking, but not too much. The bucatini will be cooked in the same water.

In the sauté, add one or two tablespoons of tomato paste, the fennel shredded with a knife, the sardines opened like a book, shredded, and carefully deprived of the bones and lateral thorns and the saffron diluted in half a glass of the cooking water of the fennel. They have been deliberately avoided: raisins, chopped almonds and pine nuts, as in the Sicilian recipe, but if desired they can be added to the sauce.

Cook the bucatini in the water of the fennel, drain very al dente and finish cooking in the sauce, diluting it, if necessary, with the same cooking water as the fennel and pasta. In a non-stick pan, in a little oil, toast the breadcrumbs until it turns brown and spread it over the bucatini.

9) Large spaghetti with clams and scampi.

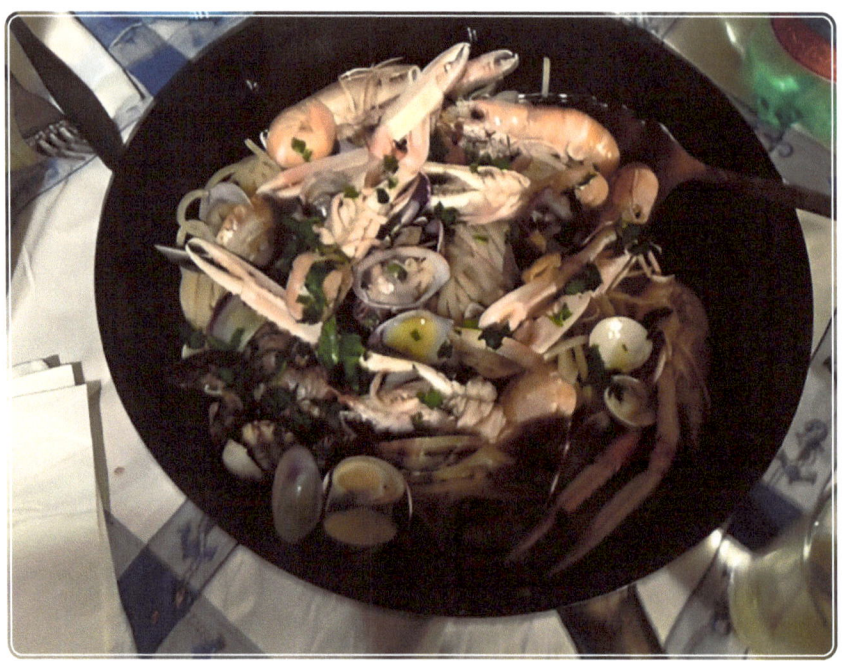

INGREDIENTS

1. 6/8 clams per person
2. 3 scampi per person
3. Parsley, finely chopped
4. Good quality dry white wine
5. 80 gr of Spaghettoni, also with egg per person
6. A sprig of rosemary
7. A piece of fresh green pepper

* The procedure of opening the fruits an oil, can also be done for spaghetti with clams, or other seafood in white and red (No for clams of the Adriatic, which express their best in white)

DIRECTIONS

Cover the bottom of a pan with extra virgin olive oil and heat the garlic.

Before the garlic turns golden, add the clams, and squeeze the heads of the scampi.
Boil the squeezed scampi heads in water and need it ready.

As the clams begin to hatch in the hot oil, add a little good quality white wine and let it evaporate quickly by raising the heat.

Remove the clams as soon as they open and the scampi tails when they turn pink and set them aside.

Shell the clams and the scampi.

Cook the pasta in lightly salted water, drain it al dente and finish cooking in the pan, adding a little water from the boiling of the prawn heads, to make the sauce creamy.

Add the clams and the scampi without their shell and sprinkle with parsley.

10) Macaroni with clams and razor clams.

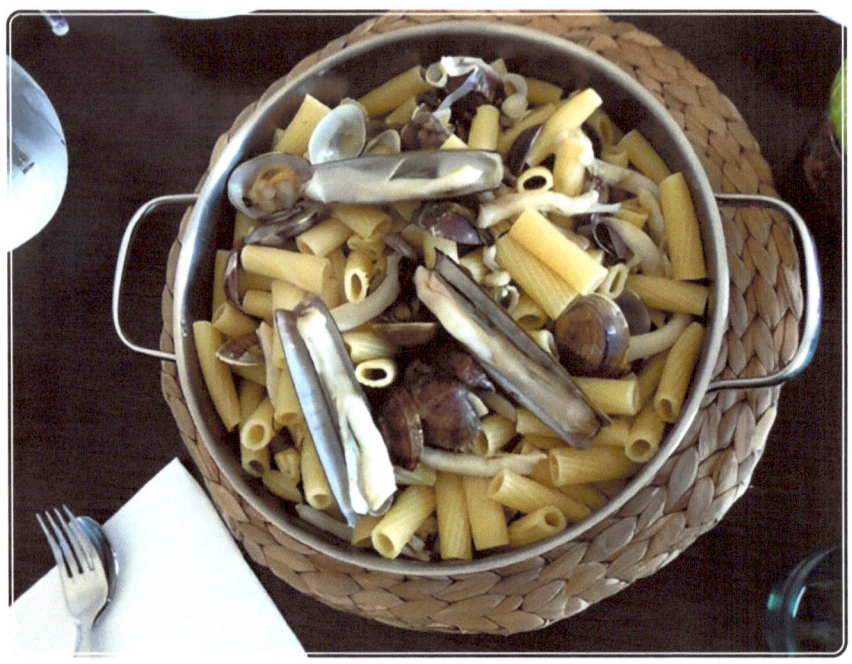

Clams and razor clams fall in love immediately.

The process for dressing is the same as recipe 9. Clams can be replaced with with large size sea clams (Paparazze) from the Adriatic.

* The procedure of opening the fruits an oil, can also be done for spaghetti with clams, or other seafood in white and red, but not red for clams of the Adriatic, which express their best in white sauce.

11) Linguine with fillets of goatfish soup.

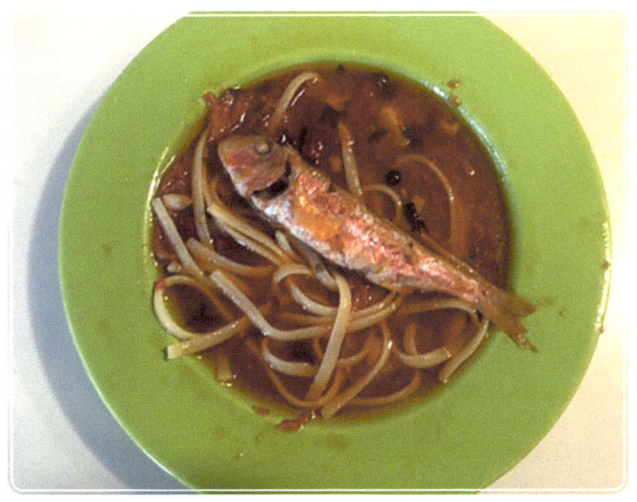

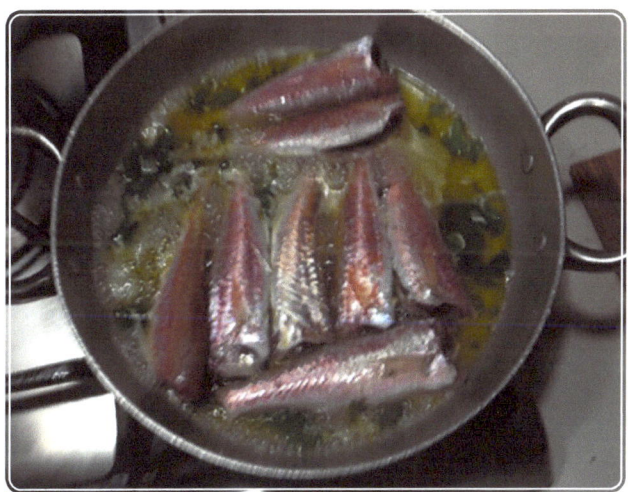

INGREDIENTS

1. 2/3 Goatfish per person
2. 300 gr of fresh tomato pulp, for the red version
3. Garlic, oil, chopped parsley, salt and pepper
4. 80 grams of quality linguine per person

DIRECTIONS

Put the oil, garlic, chopped parsley and tomato pulp in a saucepan.

Cover with salt water and bring to a boil.

Over a very low heat, reduce the broth until the oil comes up to the surface.

Add the clean goatfish whole and cook them in the broth until the eyes are white and firm.

Remove the goatfish and fillet them carefully.

Start cooking the linguine in very little salted water, as if you were cooking risotto, or covered flush with water.

Drain linguine as soon as they begin to cook and finish cooking them directly in the goatfisht broth.

Add the goatfish fillets and more finely chopped parsley on the pasta.

12) Rice with fish fillets and seafood.

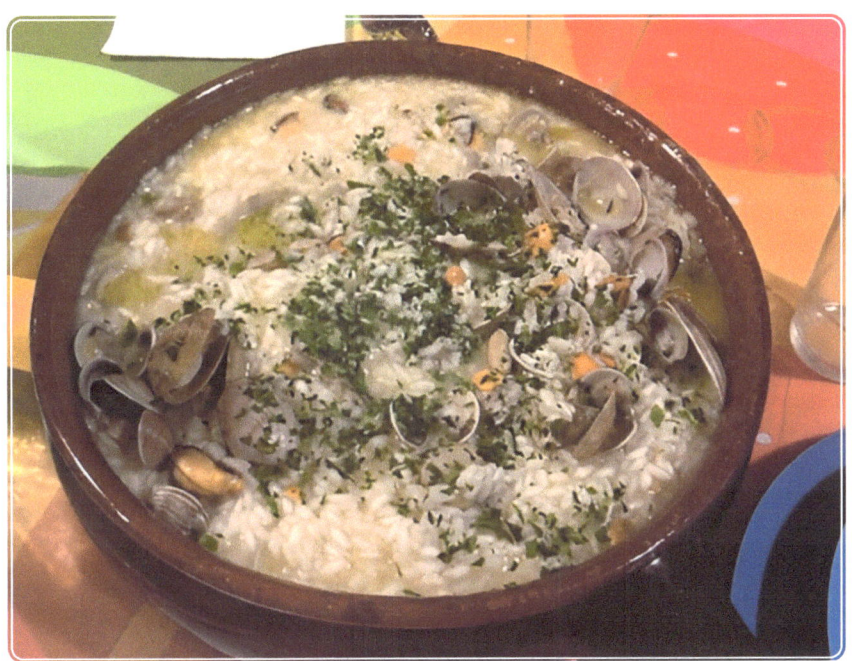

INGREDIENTS

1. Quality fish: ray, sole, monkfish, cod and other fish.
2. One bag of clams and one bag of mussels
3. A Pachino tomato every 4 people
4. Oil, garlic, spicy green pepper
5. A glass of Prosecco Brut
6. A strip of fresh green pepper
7. Quality rice for risotto, Carnaroli, or equivalent
8. Parsley, finely chopped

DIRECTIONS

Cover the bottom of a pan with extra virgin olive oil and brown the garlic cloves and a piece of onion, if desired.

Add the chopped tomatoes, which do not have to color the rice, so there will be very few.

In the base, add the selected whole fish, blanch them, and remove them immediately.

Open the mussels and clams in another pan, adding a glass of water per bag.

Remove the fruits as soon as they open and shell them; their water will be a real nectar for cooking rice.

Fillet the fish you have chosen and boil the bones, heads and a tablespoon of oil in lightly salted water to prepare a court bouillon, which will be used for cooking the rice.

In the pan of the base, in sufficient oil, toast the rice for a few minutes, gradually adding a glass of good prosecco brut and making it evaporate quickly.

When the rice is toasted, add the cooking water of the fruits first, the better the water of the clams, then continue to cook the rice by adding the court bouillon a little at a time.

In the last five minutes of cooking the rice, add the fish fillets and a handful of shelled fruits, which will open into the rice.

Sprinkle with chopped parsley and serve the risotto when it stops smoking.

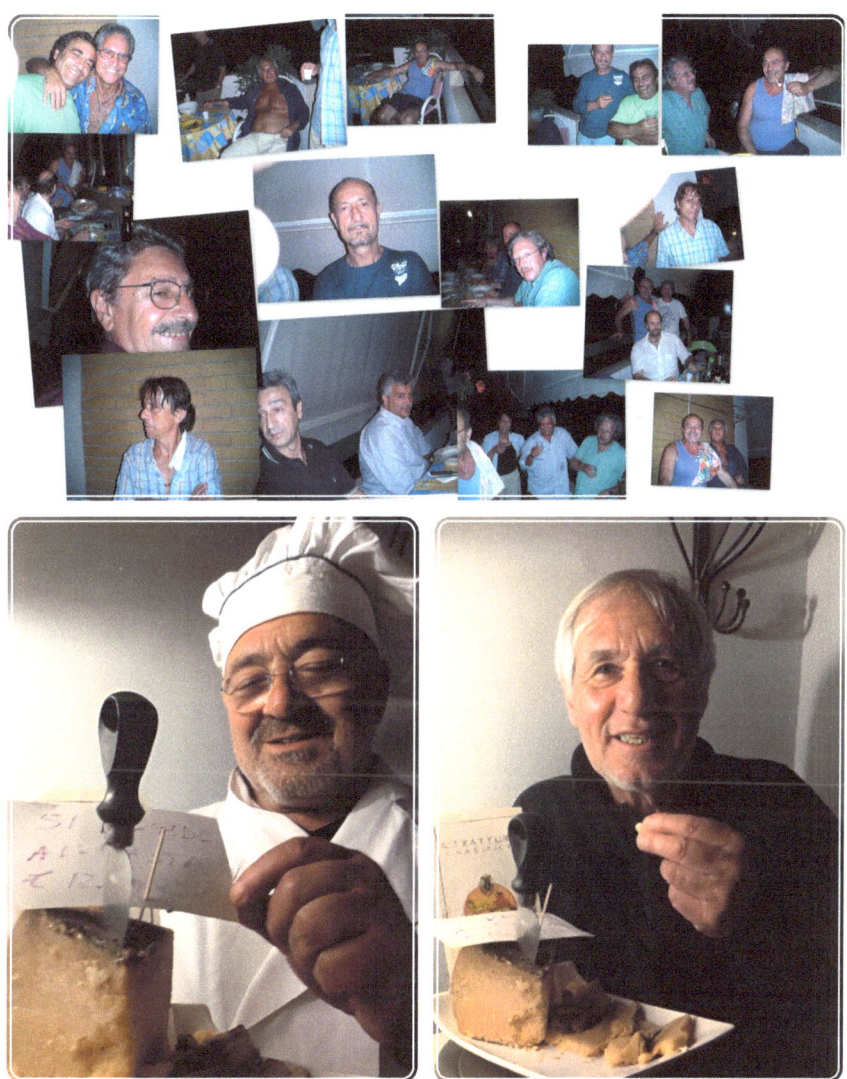

Greedy teeth meeting and drunkenness.

Gluttony & Gluttony

The fish soups perfume the landing.

Pescara style? Vasto Marina? Cooked by the fishermen on board the fishing boat?

All are worth tasting.

14) Classic fish soup from Pescara

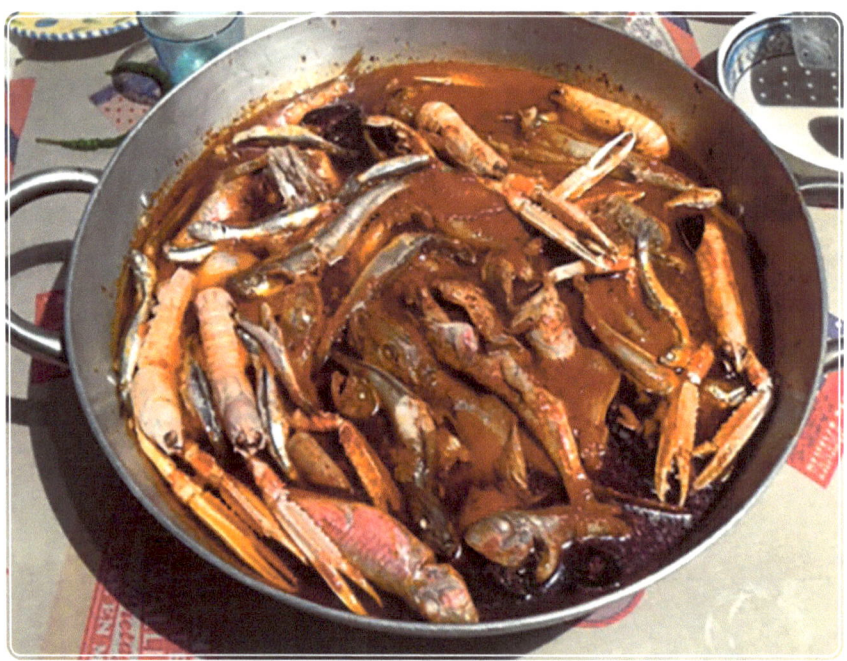

Here is the fish you need for a respectful soup.

1. Octopus, cuttlefish, squid: PRESENT!
2. Vocca'ncape (fat Head): PRESENT!
3. Ragnolo (Tracina): PRESENT!
4. Redfish: PRESENT!
5. Red mullet: PRESENT!

6. Gurnard: PRESENT!
7. Cod: PRESENT!
8. Breed piece: PRESENT!
9. Monkfish: PRESENT!
10. Panocchia (Squilla): PRESENT!
11. Scampi: PRESENT!
12. 10/12 Mussels: PRESENT!
13. 10/12 Paparazze (Lupine clams): PRESENT!
14. Any other seasonal fish.
15. Tomato puree of excellence, a strip of fresh sweet green pepper, extra virgin olive oil, garlic, fresh green or dry red-hot pepper and salt.

Do not say.

  - I had a good soup and didn't spend much. -

You didn't pay much because it was only a fake fish soup.

EQUIPMENT

An earthenware pan is preferable to an aluminum one; modern frying pans with Teflon bottoms, in other words petroleum, not even talking about it, especially if they are the cheap ones that when scratched, give up the coating.

The bottles of tomato sauce made at home in the month of August and stored in the garage, or in the closets, which are part of the Abruzzo tradition and are precious. The custom, born in the countryside to preserve tomatoes, soon spread to the city. Except for those who, for various reasons of time, cost or other, had to surrender to canned tomatoes, in almost all Abruzzo families it is rare not to find homemade tomato bottles.

DIRECTIONS

In the earthenware pan, large enough so that the fish does not overlap, put an excellent extra virgin olive oil, Abruzzo abounds with this gift of nature and if you are not stingy, that is, you do not try to save on oil, it is of excellent quality, but paying the right amount.

The amount of oil will be enough to cover the bottom of the pan with a veil, without exaggerating.

One / two cloves of Sulmona red garlic will brown in oil in the company of a couple of strips of green pepper, but just a little, because if it is too much its flavor will win over that of the sauce and the fish. Woe! (*In this case it will be better to give up the fish soup and opt for "Pependoni" Pepper and eggs.*)

The first to dive into the hot oil, after removing the browned garlic, if not desired, will be the cephalopods available: squid, cuttlefish, and octopus, which will gently fry over a moderate flame for ten minutes, or less according to their size.

This is where the bottle of good tomato comes into play, or failing that, an excellent quality tomato sauce, which will cover the cephalopods and fill the pan in sufficient quantity to accommodate all the fish and will be salted with coarse salt, adjusting because the salting of the sauce will also be that of the fish.

The tomato will be brought to a boil over high heat, which will be reduced to weak as soon as the tomato starts to boil.

The cooking time of the tomato will be about thirty minutes, and the signal that we are with it will be the return to the surface of the oil in the sauce; it's time to dip the fish in the sauce.

The fish have different cooking times, therefore the order of immersion differentiated by the greater or lesser time required will be, after the cephalopods have been browned, as follows:
I big head fish II scorpion fish, III weever, IV monkfish, V ray, VI gurnard, VII cod, VIII goatfish, IX scampi, X slipper lobster, XI, mussels and clams.

Arrange the fish so that they do not overlap in the pan and bring everything back to a light boil. After five minutes try the sauce and adjust with salt if necessary.
Never touch the fish, possibly only rotate the pan on the fire.
Add a handful of mussels and clams, not too many, otherwise they will water down the sauce.

The signal that the soup is ready will be given by the fish's eyes coming out, which when cooked become firm white balls.

According to preferences, the ways to taste this dish can be:
    A. Serve fish and sauce on some toasted slices of home-made bread.
    B. Eat the fish first, leaving enough sauce to season the bucatini.

If you like, never forget the seasonal green Abruzzo chili, or dry red flame roasted, or in a little hot oil.

14) Vasto Marina-style fish soup (Brodetto alla Vastese)

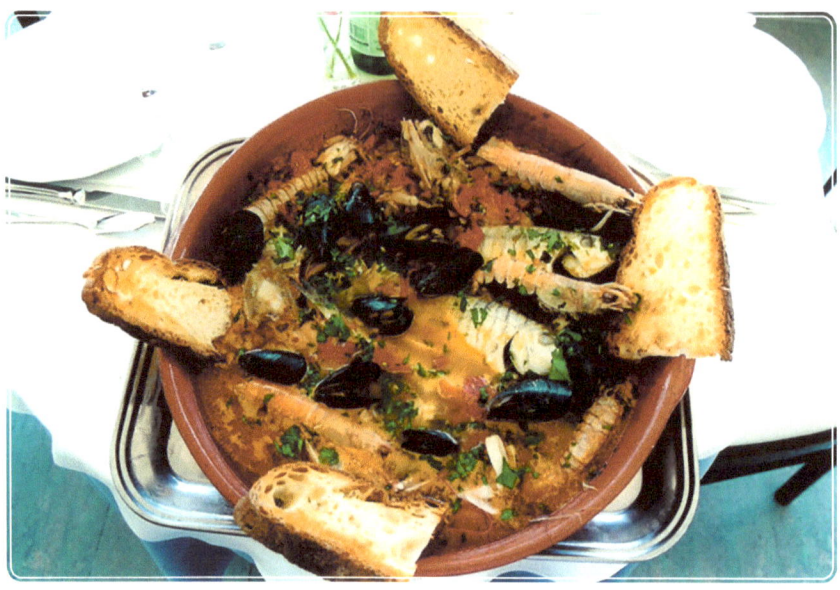

The main difference with the classic fish soup, where the tomato bottle is predominant, consists in the use of fresh tomato, chopped parsley, fresh green pepper, sweet and spicy and toasted bread, for the rest, fish and procedure are the same, even if cooking is faster.

15) Soup fish (Brodetto) with dry sweet red peppers (fishermen's from Pescara recipe)

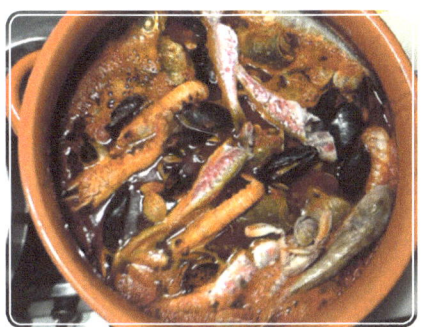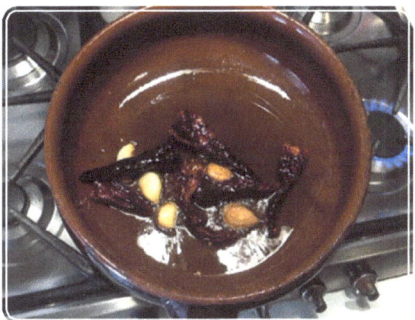

Browning in olive oil of dried red peppers; one per person.

It is the way of cooking fish on board the fishing boat using the fish of the last catch. Fishermen prefer it for its freshness and distinguish it from the one caught in the first catch, around 11.30 pm.
At lunch time, the cook on board chooses the quantity sufficient for the crew from the freshest fish, that of the last catch, and cooks it according to a procedure typical of the fishermen of the Borgo Marino di Pescara.

DIRECTIONS

The fish are those of the classic Pescara brodetto recipe 5) but the tomato sauce in the bottle is mixes with "fufulloni" *(sweet peppers dried in the sun)*, toasted in hot oil, and crashed in the mortar. Furthermore, when the *brodetto* is cooked on board the fishing boat, there are usually no mussels and clams.

The oil abounds in the pan, where three, four, "fuffulloni" and in any case no more than one every two people are toasted together garlic and spicy red pepper, otherwise the flavor of the peppers would predominate in the sauce.

Particular attention is required at this stage, because if the oil gets too hot, it starts to smoke and burns, so it will be better to remove and put the pan back on the heat, while toasting the peppers until they brown, without blackening and burning them.

As soon as they are well toasted, the peppers are removed from the oil and left to cool, salting them lightly. The expedient of keeping them in the freezer for about ten minutes will make them much more crunchy and easier to pound in the mortar, a little oil of the base sauce will be added to get a thick mixture.

The cephalopods, a nice octopus, or a squid, are usually fried first on board and when they are colored, the tomato preserve is added, that is the tomato paste that was once used to make the sauce and that was bought from the grocer of the neighborhood, wrapped in greaseproof paper. Today available in the double concentrated variant.

As soon as the preserve is amalgamated in the oil with the cephalopods, the mixture of "fuffulloni" pounded in a mortar is added with enough hot water to cover fish. Then the sauce is salted.

When the water recedes, the sauce will be ready to cook the fish which will be dipped, according to its consistency, as in the order of recipe five.

Then spaghetti *perciatelli, or bucatini*, "li brecciatelle" as they are called by the fishermen from Pescara will be seasoned with the sauce.

16) Bucatini with brodetto sauce with "fuffulloni"

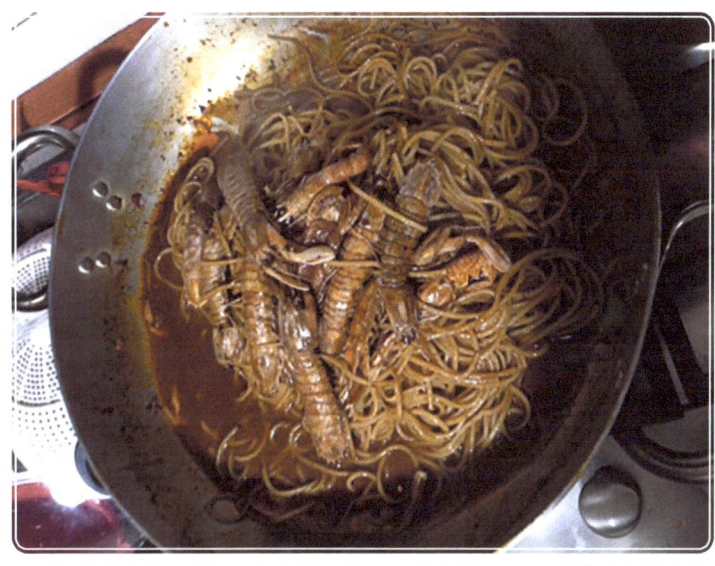

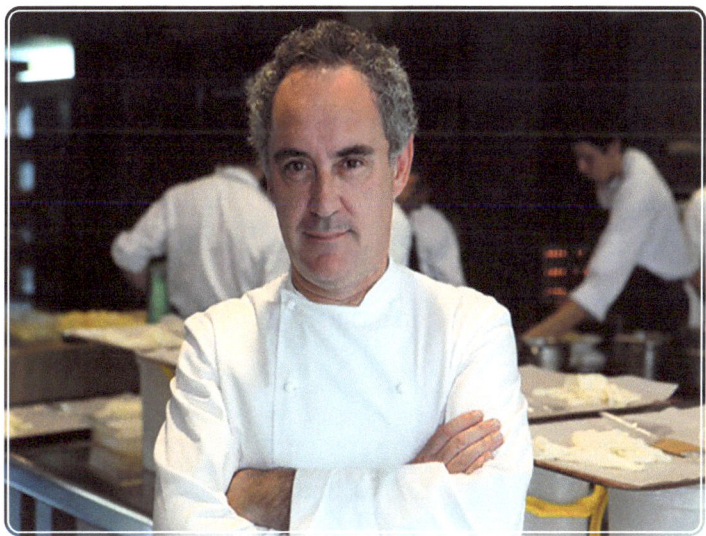

- Would please tell me the recipe? -

The great chef Adrià Ferran would have asked.

Light cooking does not mean just hospital like meal, but also delicacy.

17) Classic white soup fish
Monk fish cooked in the hunter's way.

Basically, it is fish in a white soup, where the oil must be the master. The procedure is that of the classic fish soup, without tomato. Some potatoes boiled in the fish sauce will make it a delicious dish.

INGREDIENTS

1. A gutted and skinned monkfish with the head. *(any other white fish will do)*
2. Enough oil to veil the bottom of the pan.
3. Garlic, rosemary
4. White wine of excellent quality.

DIRECTIONS

In the pan, or saucepan, put the dressed garlic, the rosemary and the monkfish in the oil and salt delicately.

Bring to a boil and wait because the monkfish releases a lot of water when cooking.

When the fish stops releasing water and begins to sizzle, add some white wine.

Let the wine evaporate, cover the pan and finish cooking the fish over low heat.

If you like you can season some spaghetti with this white fish sauce.

- God bless potatoes in white fish sauce! -

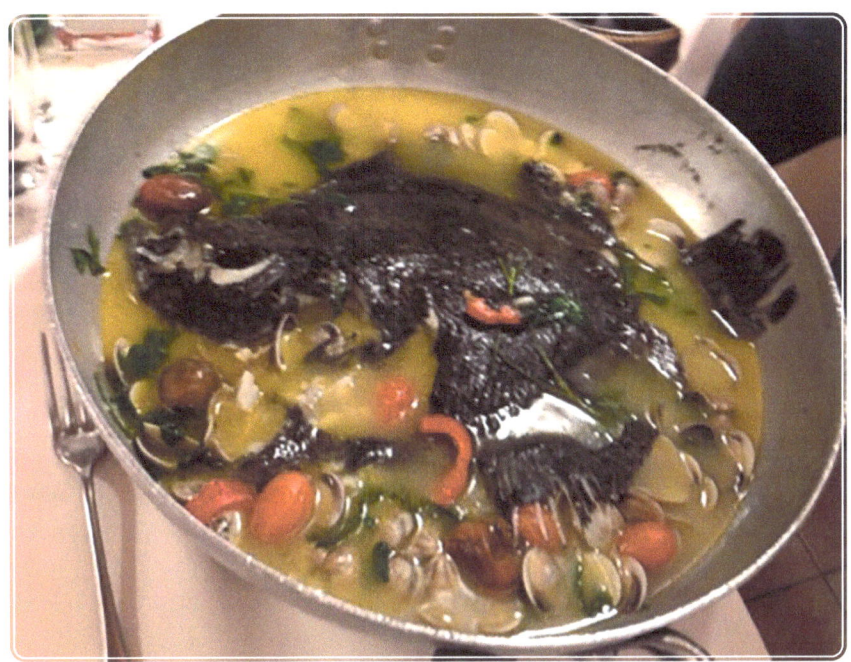

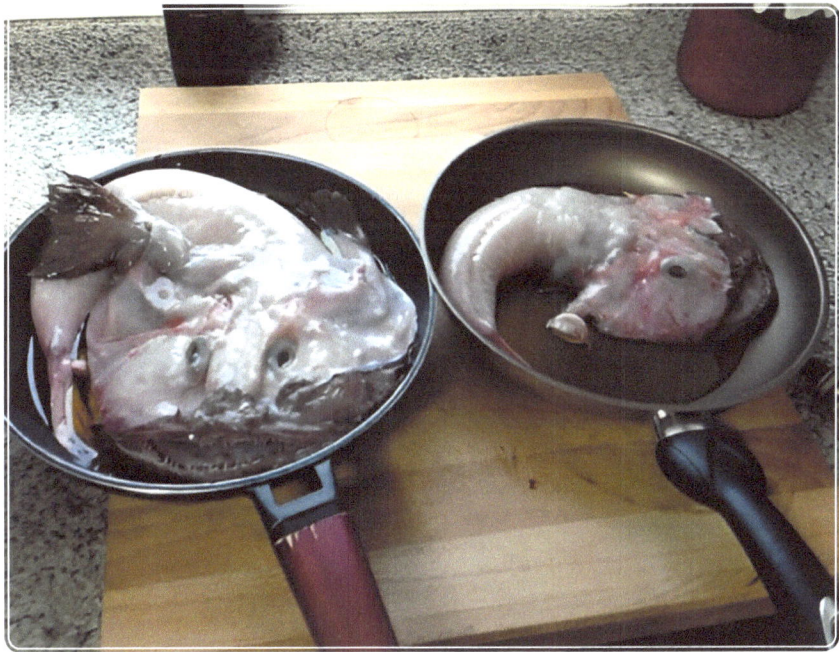

18) Scampi and potatoes

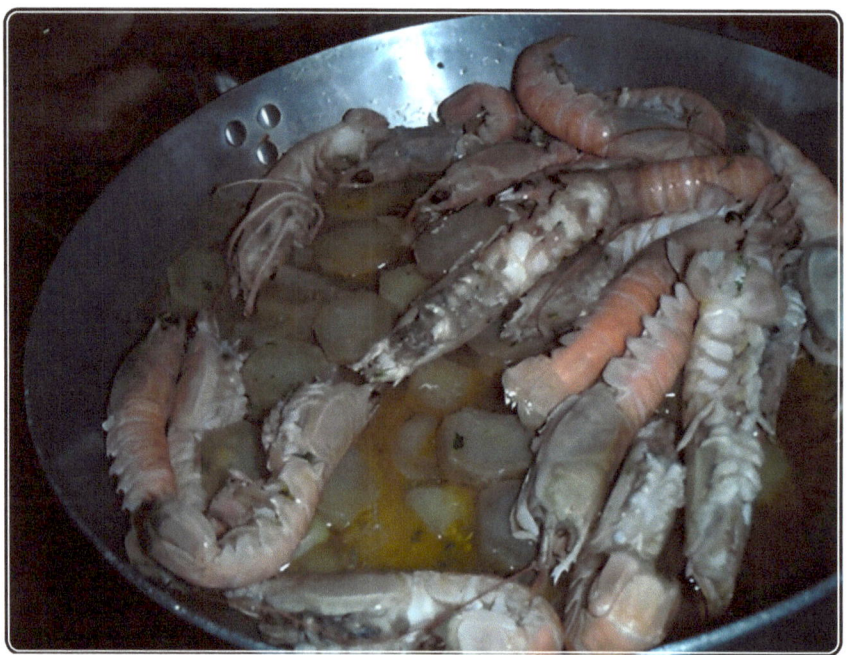

Towards the delicacy

INGREDIENTS

1. One potato per person
2. 2/3 scampi per person
3. Half a glass of quality white wine
4. Oil, garlic, and parsley
5. Spicy green chili, if dry red one is missing
6. Some chopped green pepper
7. A spring of rosemary

DIRECTIONS

Veil the bottom of the pan with high quality extra virgin olive oil.

Brown the garlic and add the spring of rosemary and the chopped red pepper.

Put in the oil the potatoes cut into slices half a centimeter thick and when they begin to fry add the wine and let it evaporate immediately.

Spring with chopped parsley, cover the potatoes with water and salt the mixture.

Cook the potatoes until they start to become tender, but do not too much.

Add the scampi and cook them with the steam emanating from the potatoes when covering the pan.

The difficulty of this dish lies in the attention needed to synchronize the cooking of the scampi at the last minutes of cooking of the potatoes.
(The recipe is by a well-known restaurateur of the Marina di Pescara, Enio Mazza.)

The dish is also excellent with "panocchie" (Silla) or prawns.

19) Tribute to the "Vocca'ncape" (Testone fat head fish)

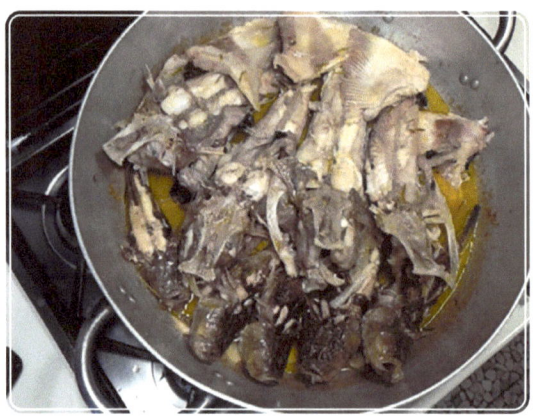

Mr. Vocca'ncape, you're already very good on your own, but now let's try to make you taste better, in good company.

INGREDIENTS

1. A good size fat head fish per person.
2. A small monk fish per person.
3. A handful of clams from Adriatic Sea
4. Oil, dressed garlic, a spring of rosemary and white wine

DIRECTIONS

The game cooking procedure is the same as recipe eighteen, but without potatoes; it differs only by the addition of a handful of clams, which with their liquid will make the fish even tastier.

Of course, a forkful of spaghetti in the basic sauce after eating the fish, will be very good

20) Small monk fish and cherry tomatoes

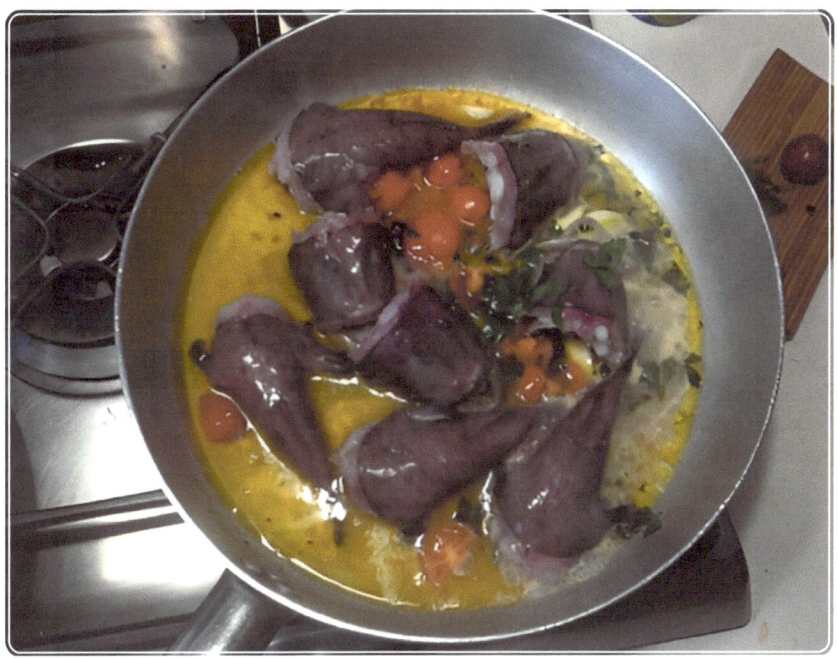

Rosé variant with small monk fish tails. Delicious with pappardelle. Large egg Noodles pasta.

Cephalopods and surroundings

21) Galician-style octopus (Pulpo à Feira)

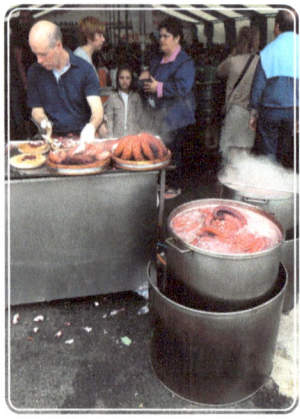 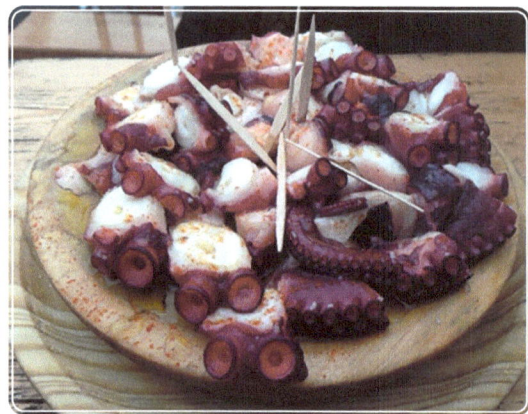

An Italian-Spanish debate on how to cook octopus. The fact is that to our best Mediterranean octopus certainly excellent Spain replies with its delicious and tender Atlantic octopus. The "Pulpo à Feira" is the typical dish of Galicia, originally served in fairs together with the Churrasco. Today the dish is a must to taste in any Galician restaurants.

INGREDIENTS

1. An Atlantic octopus of at least one and a half kg. Frozen is better because it is already crushed and softened. This type of octopus can be purchased in supermarkets that sell frozen foods.

    Fresh can only be consumed if made tender after beating them vigorously. (On board the fishermen soften them by slamming them hard many times on the deck floor.)

2. Half spoonful or more large salt.
3. extra virgin olive oil
4. Sweet, or spicy paprika

DIRECTIONS

Bring to a boil enough water to soak the octopus. Never salt the water otherwise, the octopus will harden.

When the water boils, dip the octopus three times, and then immerse it completely.
Cook the octopus for about 45 minutes and in any case until it is very tender.

Remove the octopus from the cooking water and cut the tentacles into small pieces.
Salt with medium coarse ground salt, put the oil, paprika and some cooking water.
Serve the octopus on a wooden plate.
With the "Pulpo à Feira" you should not drink red wine, but only white, so they say in Galicia.

22) Octopuses and mussels; 23) Octopuses, squillas and potatoes.

Octopus, mussels, and potatoes have always loved each other.

INGREDIENTS

1. One small octopus per person.
2. 6/7 mussels per person.
3. 200 gr of tomato pulp and two, three tablespoons of canned
4. One potato per person, for recipe 23.
5. Some spoonsful of extra virgin quality olive oil, one, or two cloves of garlic, half an onion.
6. A tablespoon of canned tomato.

DIRECTIONS

After browning the onion and garlic, put the desired cephalopods and brown them over medium heat, without frying.

Add the spoonful of preserves of tomato and mix it with the cephalopods for five minutes, turning the mixture thickly.

Add the chopped potatoes (for recipe 23), cover them with the tomato sauce and salt.

You can also choose not to put the tomato sauce to have a white version; in this case the potatoes should be covered with little hot water.

Before the potatoes finish cooking, add the mussels and any other fruits with the shells.

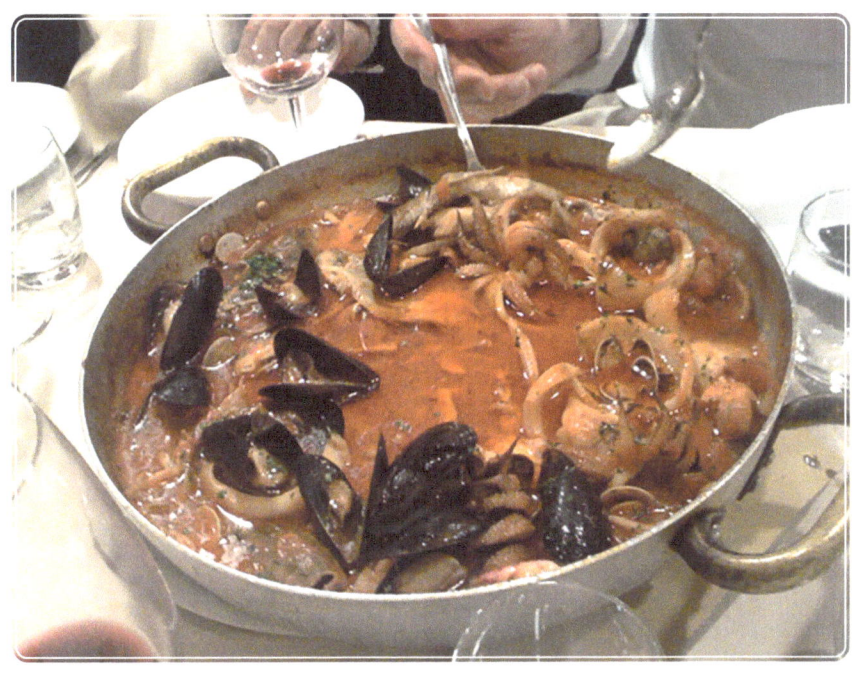

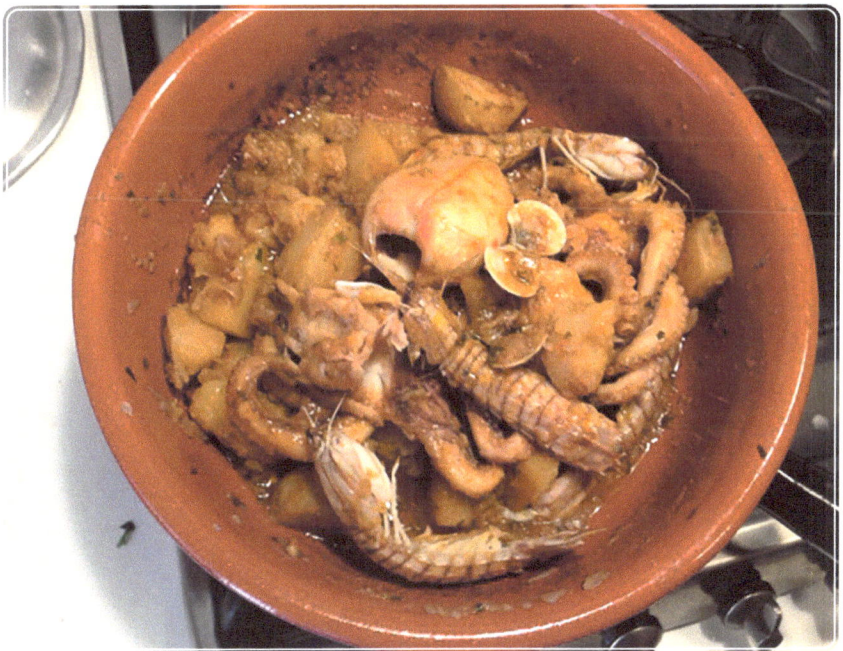

24) Mix Cephalopods cooked in a pot in the old way.

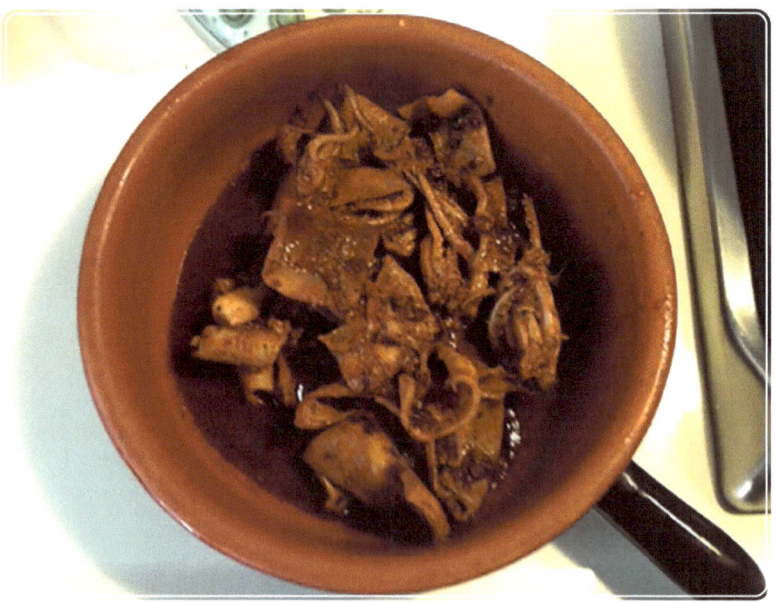

The old aunt was quite right:

> - An excellent and complete meal made of pasta as a first dish and octopus as a second. -

INGREDIENTS

This is an ancient way of cooking all types of cephalopods in a clay pot.

1. A cephalopod of your choice per person.
2. Enough oil to veil the bottom of the pot.
3. 3/4 "Fuffulloni" (Sweet red peppers, dried in the sun.)
4. A spicy red pepper, and a couple of cloves of garlic.
5. A spoonful of tomato paste.

DIRECTIONS

In hot oil with garlic, toast the dried sweet peppers, as in recipe 16 of Pescara Fishermen fish soup.

Add the chosen cephalopods and mix it with them.

Crush in a mortar the toasted sweet red peppers and it in the pot.

Pour a little hot water, as cephalopods lose a lot of liquid it during cooking and salt the sauce.

The sauce is delicious for dressing pasta.

My way

25) Monkfish tripe

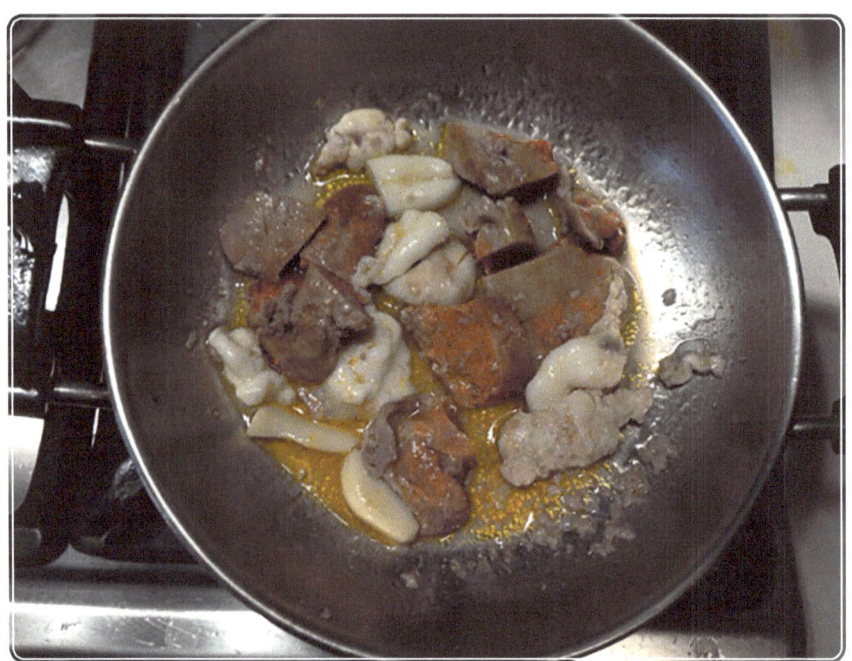

INGREDIENTS

1. One or more monk fish entrails; difficult to find, since the fishermen remove on board the monk fish gut, being a real delicacy, the sealer keep it for themselves.
2. Oil, garlic a spring of rosemary and a little white wine.
3. The oil of the dried sweet peppers toasted and crashed in a mortar.

DIRECTIONS

Quickly, given its delicacy, put the tripe in the hot oil where the garlic has become brown.

Add the rosemary and cook the tripe for a few minutes.

Add a teaspoon of oil of the battered pepper mixture and salt the sauce.

26) fresh anchovy carpaccio

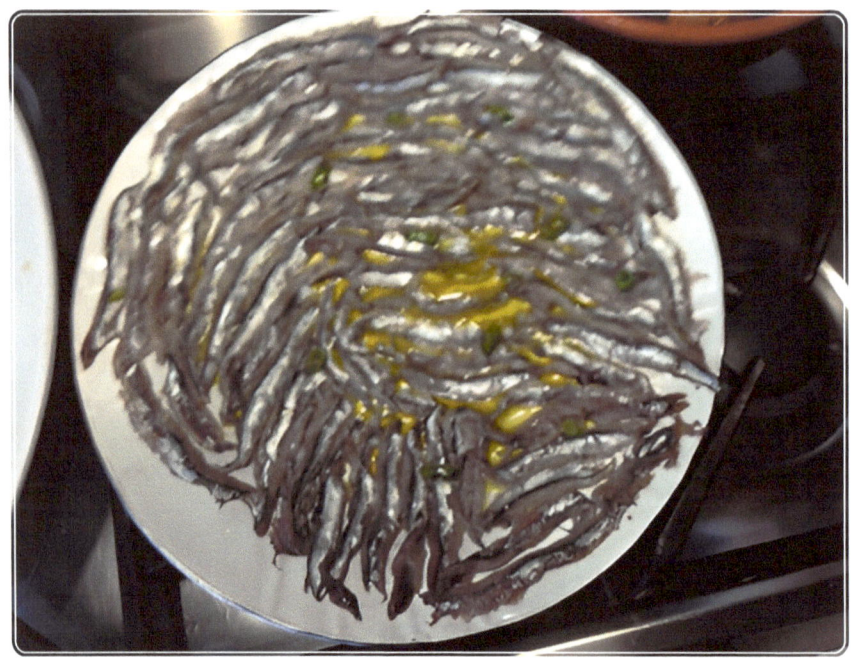

This delicious dish is often ruined by the adding of too much vinegar, which strangle your throat.

INGREDIENTS

1. 50 gr of fresh anchovies of good size per person
2. Extra virgin olive oil, garlic, salted capers, lemon

DIRECTIONS

The well-founded fear of the terrible parasite of oily fish and other fish Anisakis, suggests that this parasite can be killed with rapid freezing, so that the anchovies then can be eaten raw. In this recipe the anchovies are not raw, but burned in the lemon, so it is not necessary to freeze them.

Raw anchovies must be opened headless and smooth and placed in a non-stick pan, without overlapping them.

Spray the anchovies with the juice of a lemon, which should not be too much.

Add chopped garlic and capers desalted in water.

Brush the anchovies just raising the flame and remove them as soon as they begin to turn white.

Be careful, a prolonged cooking in the lemon makes the delicate fish too soft and unpleasant.

Drain the lemon immediately, remove the anchovies from the cooking pan and dry them well.

In a serving dish put a drizzle of oil, lay the anchovies and check the salting. Add a pinch of oregano, if desired.

27) fresh mackerel carpaccio

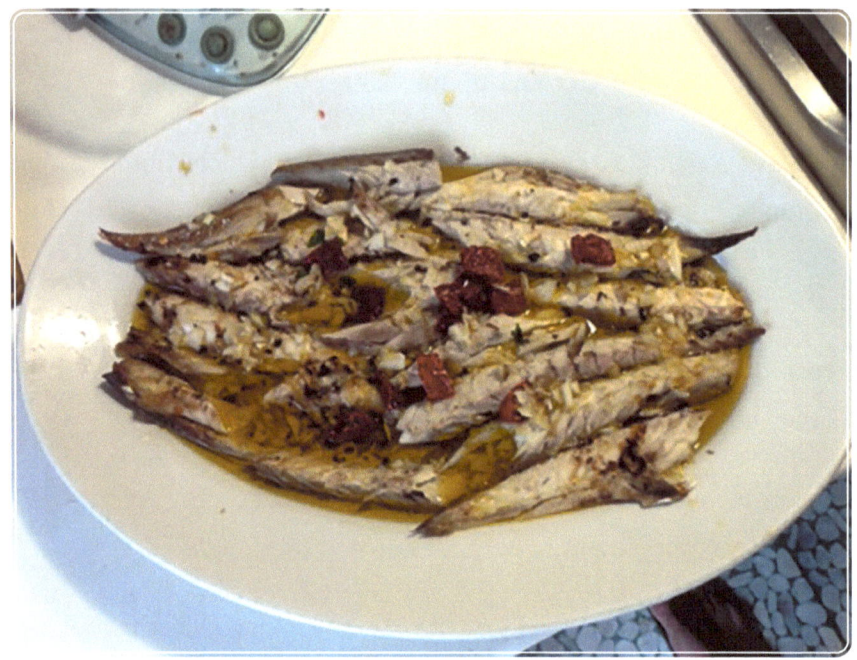

INGREDIENTS

1. One mackerel per person.
2. Half onion, 2/3 bay leaves, 3/4 grains of green pepper, vinegar, coarse salt, and white wine.
3. Extra virgin olive oil, desalted capers, oregano and green or red chili pepper.

DIRECTIONS

In a pot with enough water to cover the mackerel, put half a glass of vinegar, half a white wine, bay leaves, 3/4 grains of green pepper, half onion, and a fistful of coarse salt.

When the water boils soak the mackerel and cook them until the eyes become white and firm.

Attention, a prolonged cooking would make them soft and unpleasant.

Drain the mackerel, cool them quickly so that they harden and remove all the bones carefully.

In a serving dish put olive oil enough to veil the bottom and spread the fillets of mackerel.

Add a piece of raw thinly sliced onion, some desalted capers, a little oregano, and chili pepper.

If desired, the dressing can be colored in red, adding a little compound of crashed "fuffulloni" diluted in a spoonful of vinegar.

Sprinkle with little apple cider vinegar and check the salting, which should be tasty enough as mackerel are not.

28) fresh tuna Tartare

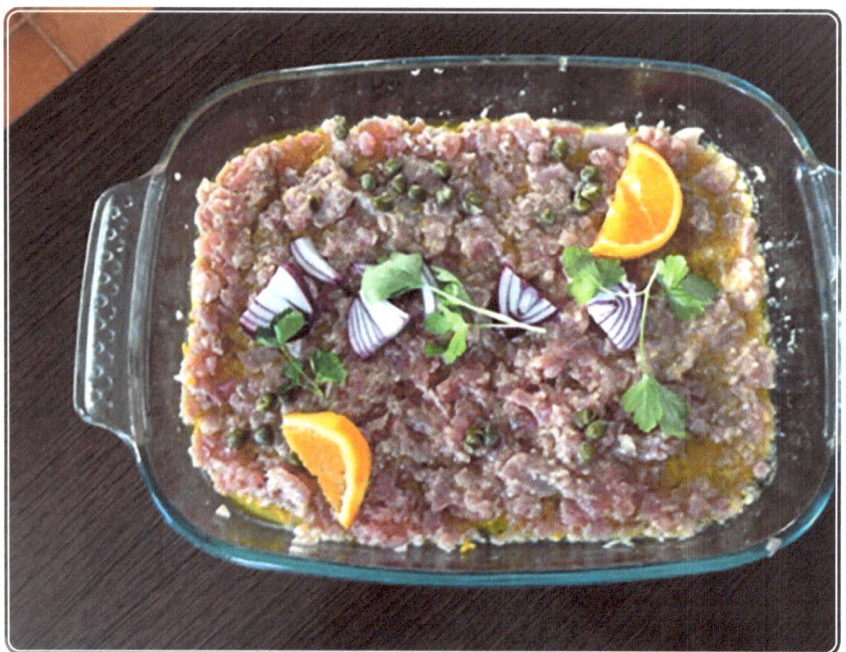

Just delicious!

INGREDIENTS

1. Defrosted red tuna fillet, 40grper person.

2. Extra virgin olive oil of the highest quality, pink salt, freshly
    ground white pepper and a few slices of orange or lime to
    decorate.

3. A few drops of green Tabasco.

DIRECTIONS

Chop the tuna into knife tip to obtain a mixture, as if it were minced meat.

Spray a terrine with oil and put the chopped tuna on it. The acidity of the good oil will cook the tuna.

Add the pink salt, a few drops of green Tabasco and the pepper.

Mix the tuna and the ingredients well with a fork and add enough oil to dress the tartare.

Check the salting and garnish with parsley leaves and slices of lime and orange.

29) Red mullet stuffed

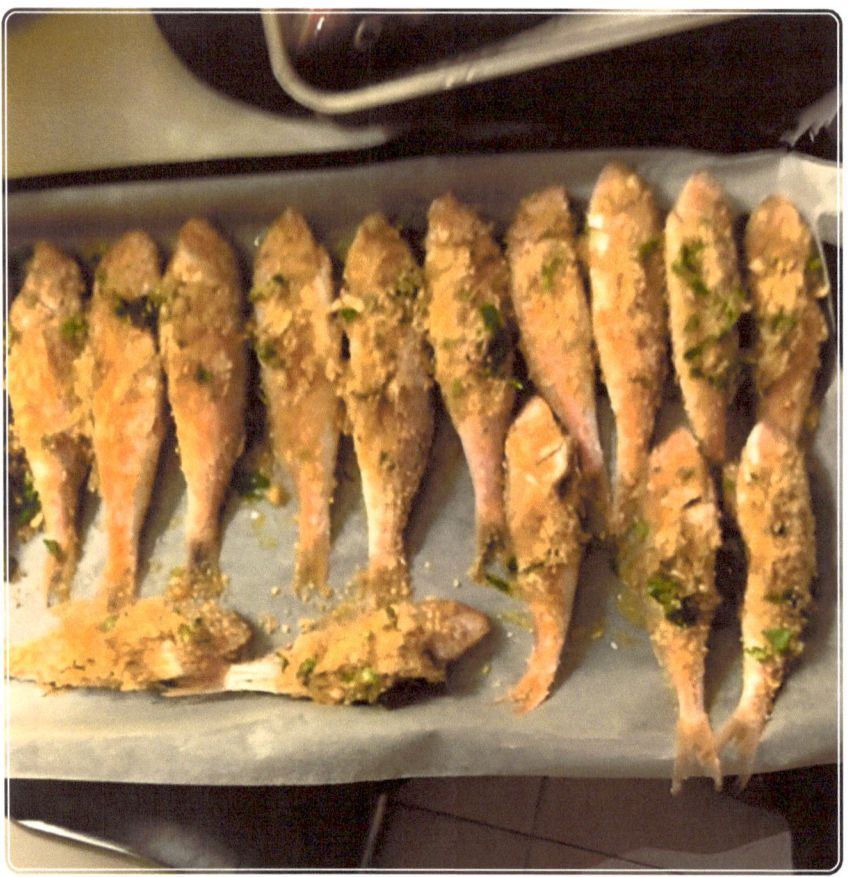

It goes on the exquisite

INGREDIENTS!

1. 3/4 fresh red mullet per person.
2. Good quality breadcrumbs, chopped oil, garlic and parsley, a strip of crushed fresh pepper and salt.

DIRECTIONS

Prepare the filling by working it in a bowl and adding the ingredients. To avoid that if it soaked too much oil, wet it with a tablespoon of hot water and then add the oil.

Regulate with salt: the filling must be tasty.

Fill the fish with the filling and bake in the oven often checking the cooking to avoid becoming too soft; 10/15 minutes at 180° and in any case as soon as the breadcrumbs begin to brown, the fish can be served.

SEA CAUGHT BASS COOKED IN SALT

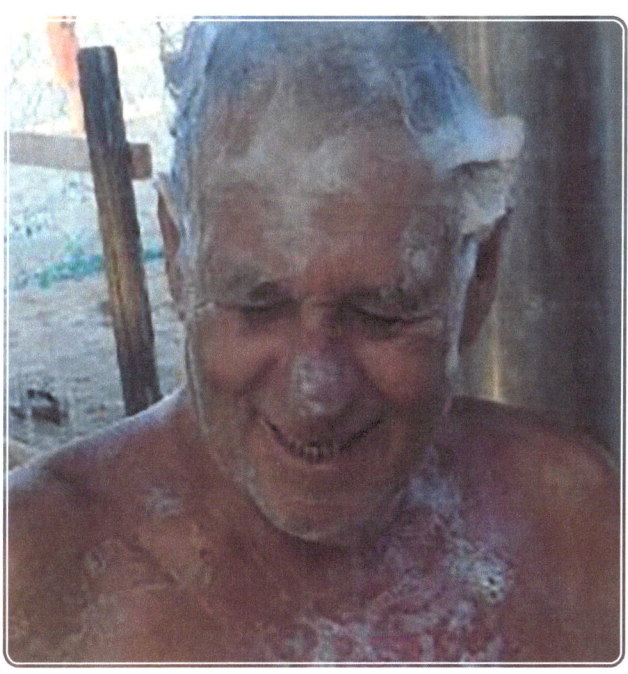

Cooked like just to please a friend.

New entry off index

30) Linguine with raw fresh tomatoes, oregano, salt capers and mussels.

The recipe comes from the search for a fresh and raw flavor.

INGREDIENTS

1. 8/12 mussels per person.
2. 300 gr of fresh raw tomato.
3. a handful of capers in salt
4. A spoonful of oregano.
5. Garlic, extra virgin olive oil.
6. Chopped parsley.
7. Hot chili pepper, if desired.

DIRECTIONS

Open the mussels over high heat and as soon as they hatch remove them, shell them, carefully filter the cooking water and keep everything aside.

In a bowl put fresh tomato pulp, deprived of seeds and skin.

Add a couple of tablespoons of oil per person, whole garlic, salted capers and oregano.

Work the sauce by adding little water of the mussels, the shelled mussels and mixing everything.

Cook the linguine in the water of the mussels, sauté them in the mixture for a few minutes cold and add the chopped parsley.

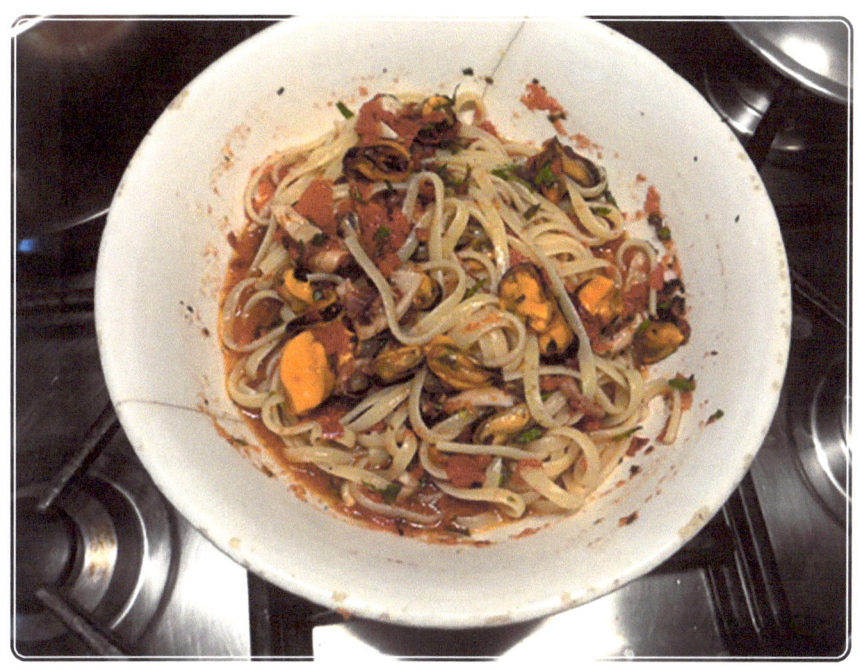

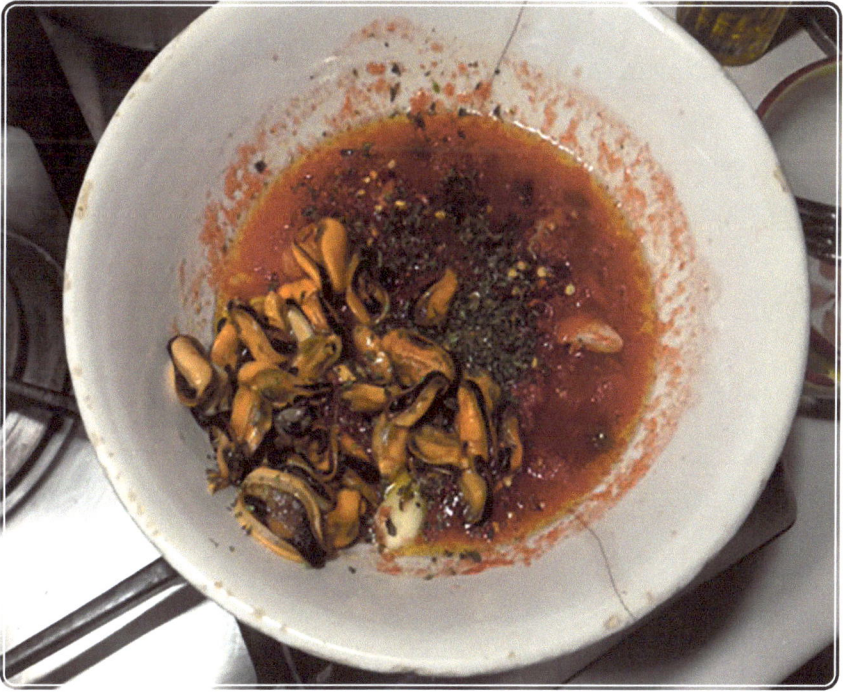

MERRY CHRISTMAS!

31) Salad Pie of December 27

Christmas and Boxing Day are gone, and all those leftovers?

INGREDIENTS

1. Advanced boiled meat of Christmas broth.
2. Vegetables from the broth.
3. Advanced meat from Pasta alla chitarra eaten on Boxing day.
4. Baked meat with potatoes, usually lamb, or turkey.
5. a handful of capers in salt.
6. Two or three boiled potatoes.
7. Dijon mustard.
8. Pickles, better if homemade.
9. Quality mayonnaise.
10. Tomato Ketchup Heinz, a few drops of Tabasco and Worcestershire Lea Perrin Sauce.
11. Some slices of lemon, and orange.

DIRECTIONS

On a wide wooden cutting board, put all the leftovers from No. 1 to No. 5.

Chop them and work them with a knife, adding a drizzle of oil to soften them.

Incorporate the crushed boiled potatoes into the mixture.

Add two spoonsful of sauce, mustard, ketchup, mayonnaise and a few drops of the above sauces.

Garnish the dish with pickles, mayonnaise and slices of lemon, or orange.

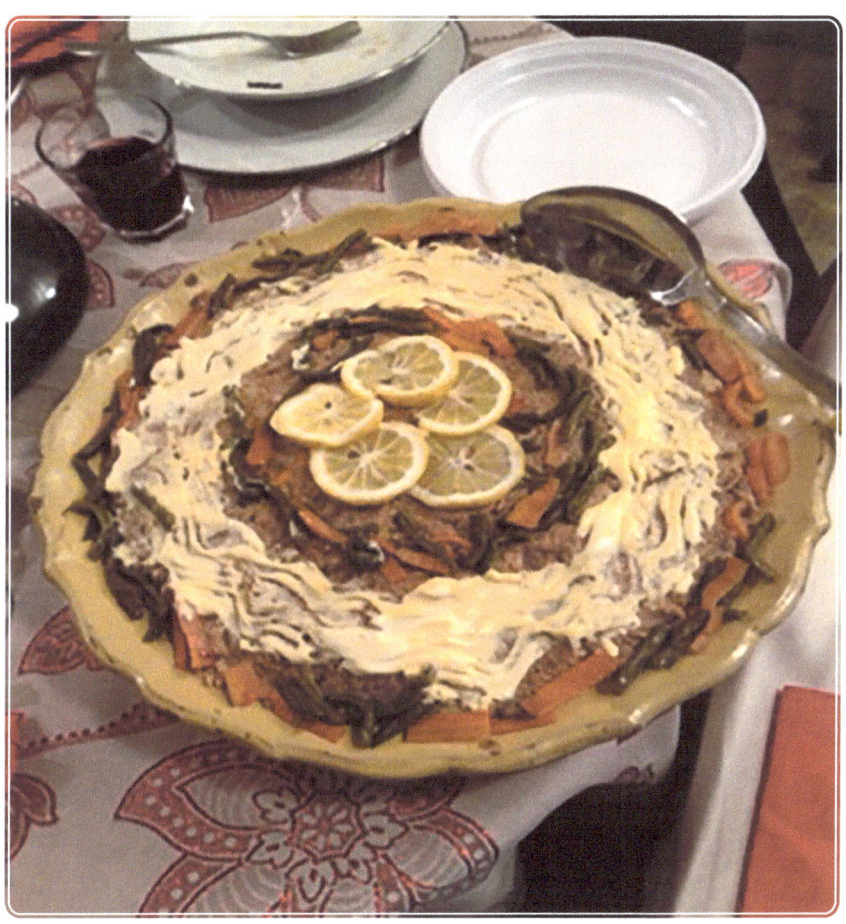

Fish is good, but "arrusticine..." *(Roasted sheep meat. Street food typical from Abruzzi.)*

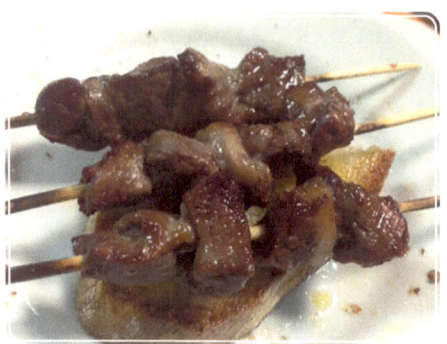

ITAGLIANI! W LABRUZZO!

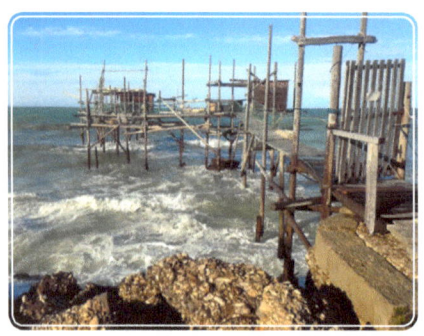

Costa dei trabocchi pissed off

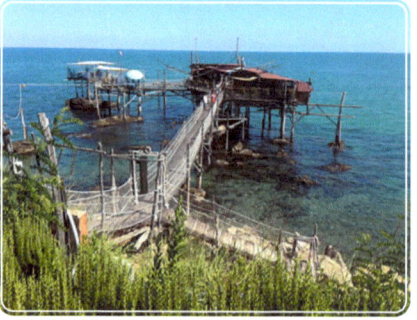

Costa dei Trabocchi realaxed

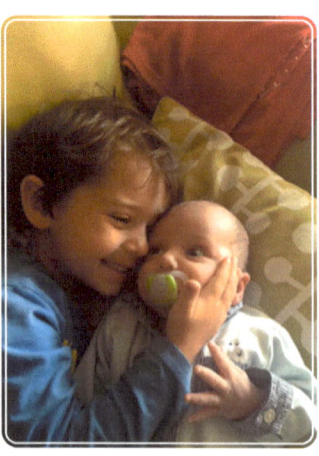

Shall I make some juicy "Arrosticini" with them?

Her Majesty PIZZA

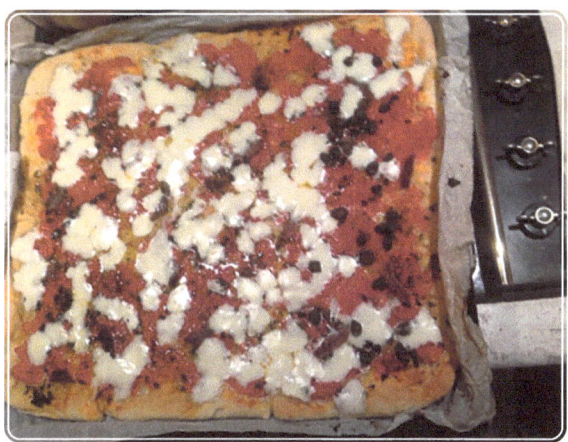

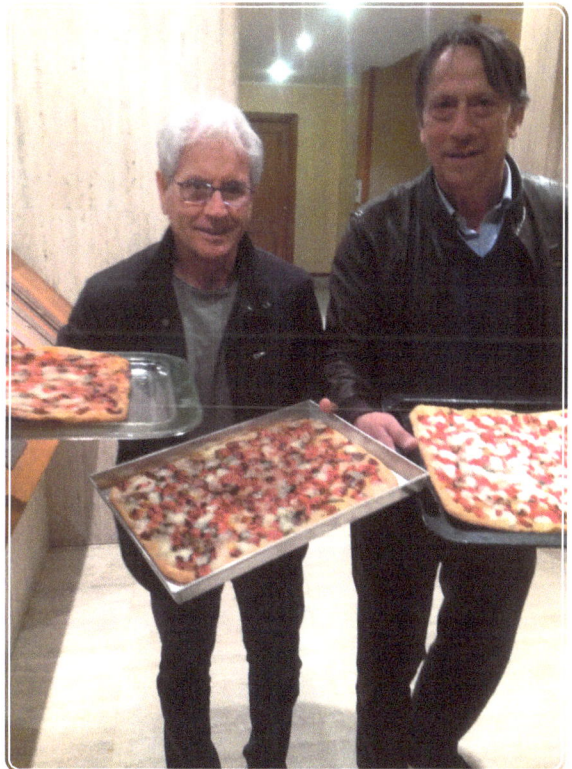

The sovereign of pizza is a certain lady who, if she had worked as a professional pizza maker, she would be a millionaire today.

And then
NOT JUST FISH

Antica Locanda del
Professor Ghiottone
Pasqua 2016
Menù

Antipasto - Salsicce abruzzesi DOC con lampacioni.

Primo - Chitarra con polpettine alla teramana. Ravioli di carne.

Secondo - Stufato di vitello al sugo. Capretto alla cacciatora. Capretto cacio e ovo. Testina di capretto gratinata. Cif e ciaf di interiora di capretto. Eccellenza di Pecorino abruzzese.

Contorni - Patate rosse. Puntarelle di cicoria in salsa. Carciofi fritti.

Dolce - Torta Giuliana

Frutta - Delicatesse Maroquine

Vini e liquori - Montepulciano d'Abruzzo Collemoro. Prosecco Muller Turgau. Fernet Branca. Gin di Galizia. Caffè miscela India Tavoletta.

Ingredienti

Salsicce teramane e lampacioni di produzione casereccia. Chitarra e ravioli artigianali senza conservanti. Capretto di Carpineto della Nora da allevamento non intensivo. Pecorino dell'azienda agricola il Tratturo di Cepagatti. Parmigiano reggiano vacche Rosse. Olio Extra vergine e salsa di pomodoro da contadini di Larino. Pane di semi integrali di Cepagatti. Caffè India a tostatura artigianale Ditta Tavoletta. Arance dall'egiziano Terra dei Fuochi e frutta esotica.

Pescara, London and Santiago de Compostela
Thank you for your attention.
To be continued…
February 2017

Some more dishes added to the first edition of the recipe book.

32) Spaghetti/Linguine with peeled scampi and seasoned anchovy juice from Cetara.

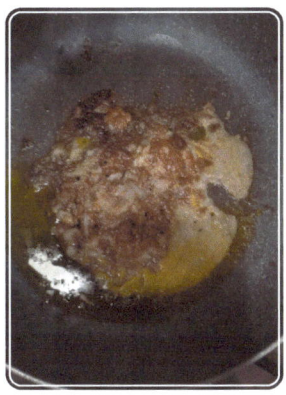 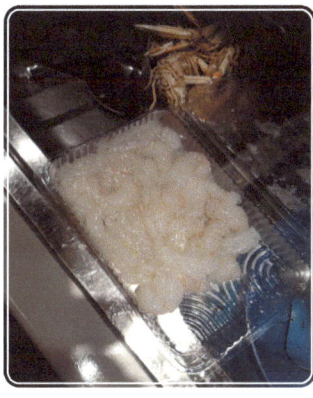 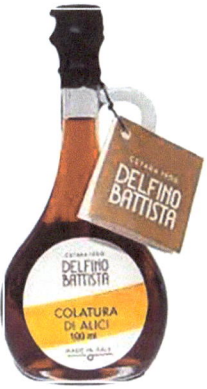

Ingredients for four people

1. 3/4 Peeled scampi per person.
2. The heads of the scampi.
3. A large quantity of finely chopped parceley.
4. One tablespoon of oil per person.
5. One tablespoon of seasoned anchovy juice from Cetara per person.
6. 2/3 tablespoons of good quality breadcrumbs.
7. An organic lemmon peel.
8. Green spicy chili, or dry red.

PROCEDURE

In a bowl, or container that will serve the pasta, put a tablespoon of oil per person, parsley, a piece of chili pepper, garlic cut in little round pieces and a tablespoon of seasoned anchovy juice from Cetara per person.

Mix everything in cold. In a non-stick pan put three tablespoons of oil, squeeze the heads of the scampi, and add them after peeling.

Heat the juice using the Bain- Maria method. Do not overheat the juice and the peeled scampi. Do not add salt to the water for cooking pasta.

In a non-stick pan toast the breadcrumbs until golden.

Cook the favorite pasta, drain it al dente, and pour it into the bowl with the mixed ingredients. Add the juice of the head of the scampi and mix well.

Sprinkle with the browned breadcrumbs. Grate some lemon peel. Put on top the peeled scampi.

Avoid any dryness of the pasta by adding some cooking liquid.

If the squeezed heads of the scampi have beautiful claws, boil, and serve them seasoned with salt pepper, and oil.

33) Spaghetti/Linguine with Adriatic clams

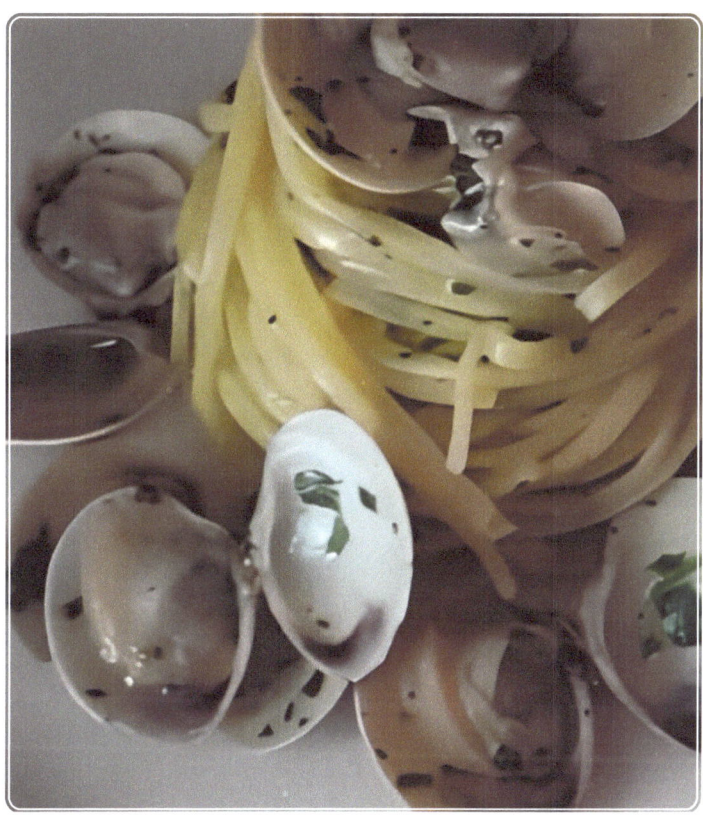

INGREDIENTS for four people

1. 1 kg of good-sized Adriatic clams
2. Spaghetti/Linguine, or home made egg pasta (Chitarra Abruzze) 400 gr.
3. Green Chili
4. Parsley
5. A clove, or two of garlic
6. Olive Oil
7. A glass of plain water for each kg o

PROCEDURE

Open the clams over high heat, after adding one glass of water for each kg of clams (The clams must purge the sand completely and must be kept in salt water for at least three to four hours, unless they are already purified.)

As soon as they hatch, remove them immediately from the heat, a prolonged cooking would harden them.

Shell the clams and filter the cooking water.

In a pan that will be used to pan-fry the pasta to and then serve it, put a tablespoon and a half of olive oil per person.

In the oil brown a garlic and a few shelled clams, a piece of green chili pepper and little parsley leaves chopped by hand.

When the garlic is golden add the filtered water of the clams.

Add a pinch of salt and the stalks of the parsley to the water for cooking pasta.

Halfway through cooking, drain the pasta, put it in the pan, and finish its cooking adding the water of the clams.

Add the shelled clams and finely chopped parsley.

If pasta is too dry add some more clams' water and a drizzle of olive oil.

34) Spaghetti/Linguine with seafood and tomato

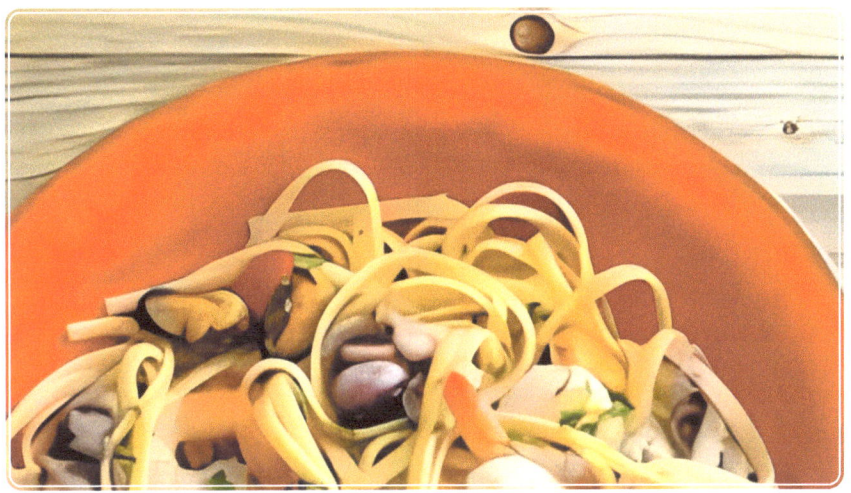

INGREDIENTS FOR FOUR PEOPLE

1. A bag of good-sized Adriatic clams
2. Alternatively, one kg of good quality mussels.
3. Spaghetti/Linguine, or guitar 400 gr.
4. Green Chilli
5. pre-packaged
6. Garlic
7. Olive Oil
8. Essential boiling water for clams.
9. Three, four ripe ox heart tomatoes.

PROCEDURE

Open the clams over high heat, after adding a glass of water. (The clams must purge the sand completely and must be kept in salt water for at least three to four hours unless they are already purified).

As soon as they hatch, remove them immediately from the heat, a prolonged cooking would harden them.

Shell the clams and filter the cooking water.
Boil the ripe tomatoes for 2, 3 minutes, and just peel them cold.

In a stainless-steel bowl put the peeled tomatoes, a tablespoon of oil per person, garlic, hand chopped parsley, a pinch of freshly ground pepper, a piece of green chili pepper and filtered water of the fruits.

Bring the mixture to the boil. In another pot cook the pasta (see cooking pasta the pasta, Recipe Book 1) and halfway through cooking frypan it into the mixture and finish cooking.

Add the fruits and the finely chopped parsley.

Serve the pasta adding a little cooking water and a drizzle of oil, in case it is too dry.

35) Marinated salmon

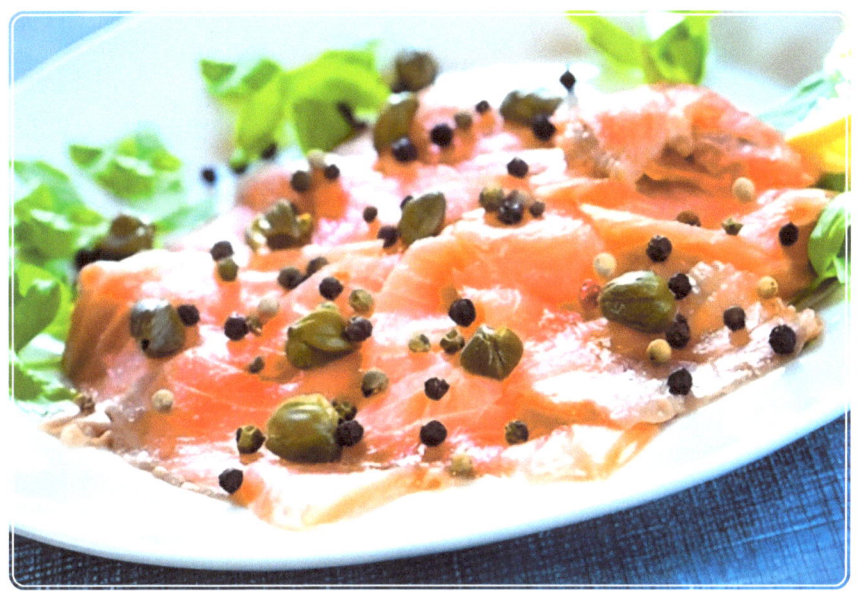

INGREDIENTS FOR FOUR PEOPLE

1. A salmon fillet of 500/600 gr, or larger
2. Sugar
3. a teaspoon of honey
4. Oil
5. Chilli pepper
6. Pepper
7. Tropea onion or Red onion
8. Lemon

PROCEDURE

Prepare a mixture by mixing one part salt with two parts sugar; use a cup, or glass to measure.

In a terrine that may contain the whole salmon fillet put a layer of the sugar and salt compound.

Lay the salmon on the side of the skin.
Cover the fillet with the mixture.

Keep everything in the fridge for 24 hours.
Rinse the salmon to remove salt and sugar.

Dry it well with kitchen towel.
Fillet the salmon into thin slices and remove the skin.

Pour oil into the basin to wet the bottom.
Place the slices in the layered oil.

Season with oil, freshly ground pepper, onion cut into thin slices and pieces of green chilli pepper.

Serve with some lemon wedges and toasted bread.

Marinating can also be done with sea bass, or with other fish.

36) Spaghetti with garlic, oil, chili, and cuttlefish (Sepia)

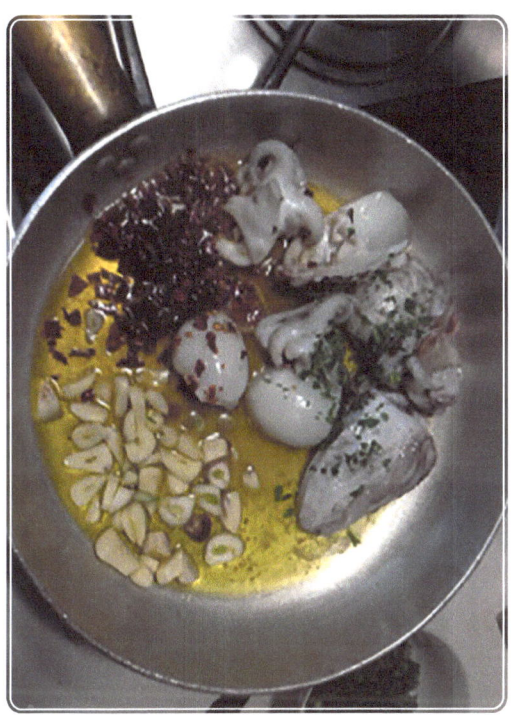

INGREDIENTS

1. 1 fresh cuttlefish (sepia) per person.
2. 3/4 cloves of garlic per person, plus 2/3 cloves for each additional person.
3. A spicy chili pepper, a pinch of salt to salt the cuttlefish.
4. A tablespoon of chopped sweet pepper (Fuffullone).
5. Quality extra virgin olive oil, just enough to veil the bottom of the pan.
6. Large spaghetti, eighty grams, or more per person.
7. A couple of tablespoons of good quality breadcrumbs.

DIRECTIONS

In a pan heat the olive oil, put the garlic cloves cut into rolls, the hot chili pepper into pieces and the sweet pepper If garlic is not liked you can decrease its quantity, but the dish will no longer be spaghetti garlic, oil, and chili pepper!

Let the garlic dusk well, toast the sweet pepper and salt the two ingredients very little. To prevent them from burning remove and put the pan back on the fire, then add the whole cuttlefish and brown them for only two or three minutes.

Remove the cuttlefish, pass them in the breadcrumbs and finish cooking on the steakhouse (Simplified procedure, the optimal would be to grill them on coals)

Cook the spaghetti, drain them al dente and finish cooking by skipping them directly into the base sauce; any dryness of the pasta and the sauce are corrected by adding some water used for cooking pasta.

37) Mediterranean-style spaghetti with raw tomato and spices

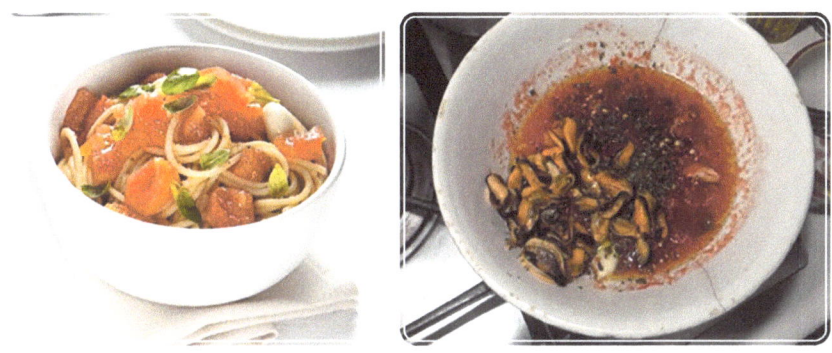

With mussels

Ingredients and quantity

1. 80 gr of spaghetti per person.
2. 2/3 tablespoons of capers desalted in running water.
3. One shallot
4. One/two cloves of garlic.
5. 3/4 anchovy fillets in oil.
6. Handful of chopped parsley
7. 3/4 pitted black baked olives.
8. A spring of rosemary.
9. 4) A spoonful of oregano.
10. Some hot pepper.
11. 1/2 ripe tomatoes per person.
12. 2 tablespoons of extra virgin olive oil per person.
13. A piece of celery heart
14. White pepper, or freshly ground green.
15. Grated Pecorino DOC from Abruzzo, if desired.

DIRECTIONS

Blanch the ripe tomatoes, peel them and let them cool in the fridge.

In a bowl large enough to hold the ingredients first, and pasta later, put the cooled tomatoes and the tablespoons of oil.

Prepare a not too finely chopped smoothie with all the ingredients listed above.

Incorporate them with the oil and the peeled raw tomato and mix the mixture.

Cook the spaghetti with a pinch of salt in the water, drain them al dente and flavor them in the mixture by mixing well.

The dish lends itself to being enriched with the addition of 4/5 mussels per person and a little cooking water of the same. (Picture on the right)

38) Spaghetti Matriciana with potato mousse

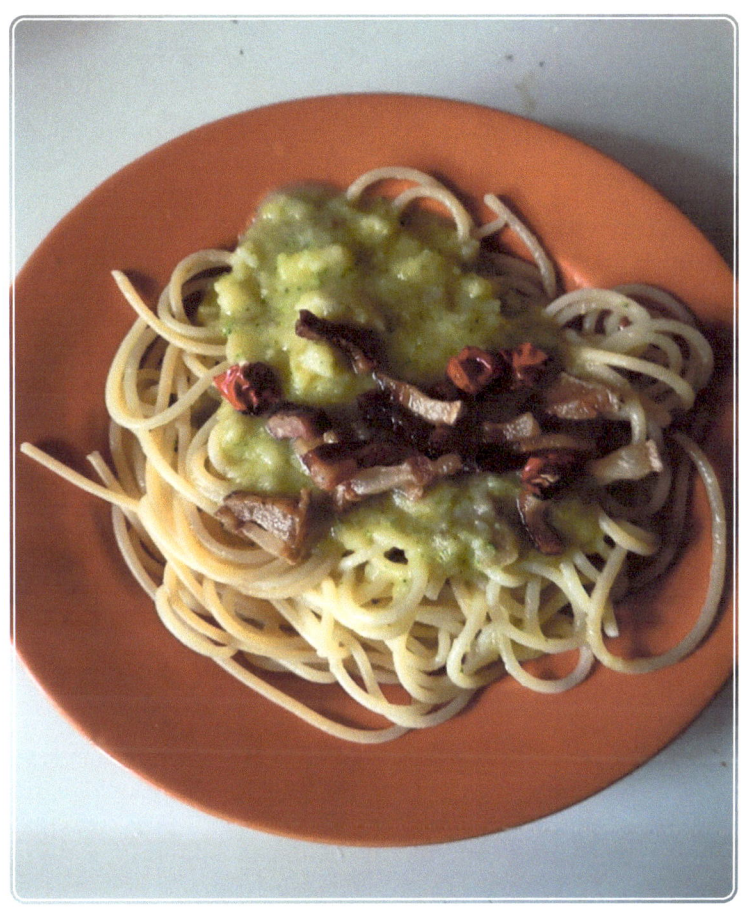

INGREDIENTS FOR ONE PERSON

1. 1 potato
2. A sprig of green broccoli
3. 40grquality fresh bacon
4. Two tablespoons of extra virgin olive oil
5. A little red chopped pepper
6. 80 gr quality spaghetti

DIRECTIONS

Boil the potato with the peel and the sprig of green broccoli in water with a pinch of salt.

In a non-stick frying pan toast the fresh bacon cut into not too small pieces, until its fat is liquefied.

Drain the toasted bacon remove its liquefied fat, drying it with kitchen towel.
In a bowl that will be used for pasta put the ingredients as it follows.

I The boiled potatoes cut into small pieces.
II The boiled green broccoli.
III The oil needed per person.
IV Salt and pepper

Chop the ingredients with the minipimer, but do not make them too liquid.
Drain the spaghetti and put them in the mixture, mixing everything well.
Add on top the toasted bacon and a little pasta cooking water.

If desired, sprinkle with a good Pecorino from Abruzzo cheese.

39) Faruk-style Pasta alla chitarra

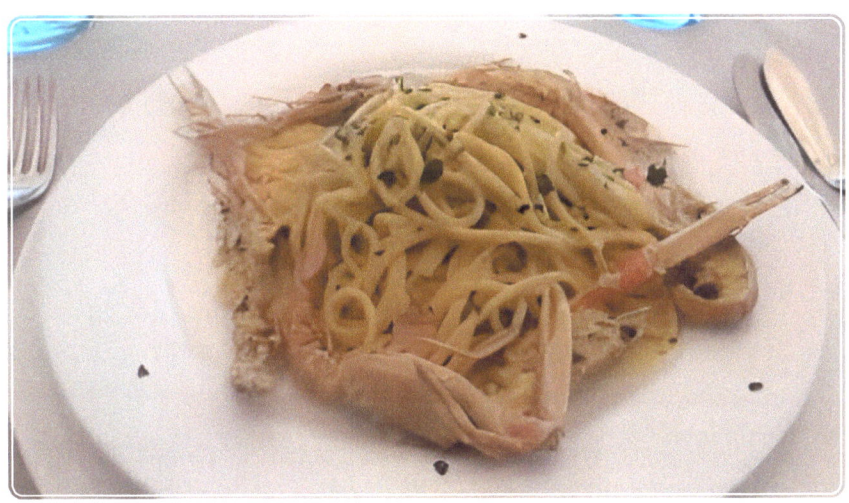

(Remake of a recipe "stolen" to a great chef, Narciso Bonetti, whom I had the pleasure to meet at his restaurant Casa Mia, famous in Abruzzo, in the seventies)

INGREDIENTS FOR FOUR PEOPLE

1. 350 gr of homemade "Pasta all'uovo alla Chitarra Abruzzese", or noodless if egg pasta is not available.
2. 16 raw shelled scampi, plus three whole four for the presentation of the dish.
3. 12 shelled mussels and three, four with the shell for the presentation of the dish.
4. The heads of the scampi
5. 16 prawns
6. One, two tablespoons of Curry, brand MIDA TRS, Hot (Spicy) or Mild (Not Spicy) available in Indian and Chinese stores. (The amount of curry depends on the taste)

7. One nut of butter for every 100 grams of spaghetti.
8. 350 cl of cooking cream, however 100 cl per 100gr of pasta.
9. Half a glass of good brandy.
10. A splash of good white wine.
11. One shallot.
12. Th juice from 1/2 lime
13. Salt, black pepper, parsley, and chili pepper in the desired quantity.
14. A small saffron bag.
15. Two Extra virgin olive oil spoonful per person.

DIRECTIONS

In a pan that then will contain the pasta, put the spoonsful of olive oil and the butter.

Add and brown the finely chopped shallots.

Add the white wine first, then the brandy until the alcohol evaporates completely.

Squeeze the scampi heads and add the liquid to the sauce.

Add the cooking cream and mix with the sauce over very low heat.

Boil the heads of the squeezed the scampi in water with a few leaves of parsley and a little salt to have a delicate Bouillon court. (The pulp of the claws, if desired, is excellent to taste separately.)

The heads of the scampi cooking
In the boiling water of the squeezed heads, stir: 1 little bag of saffron, 2 spoonsful of curry, 3 ½ lime juice.

Add the mixture to the base sauce, which must be creamy and balanced in taste of cream, butter, oil, and court bouillon.

Add the scalded and shelled mussels, prawns and finally the raw shelled scampi to the sauce that will turn yellow because of saffron and curry.

Check the salting and add a little ground pepper.

Always keep the pan with the sauce on low heat, never let it cool. Drain the pasta very al dente and finish cooking by stirring it in the sauce.

Garnish the dish with scampi, open mussels, some shrimp, and finely chopped parsley.

The Abruzzese chili is at your discretion because it could be in contrast with the spicy Curry.

40) Linguine with salt cod fish

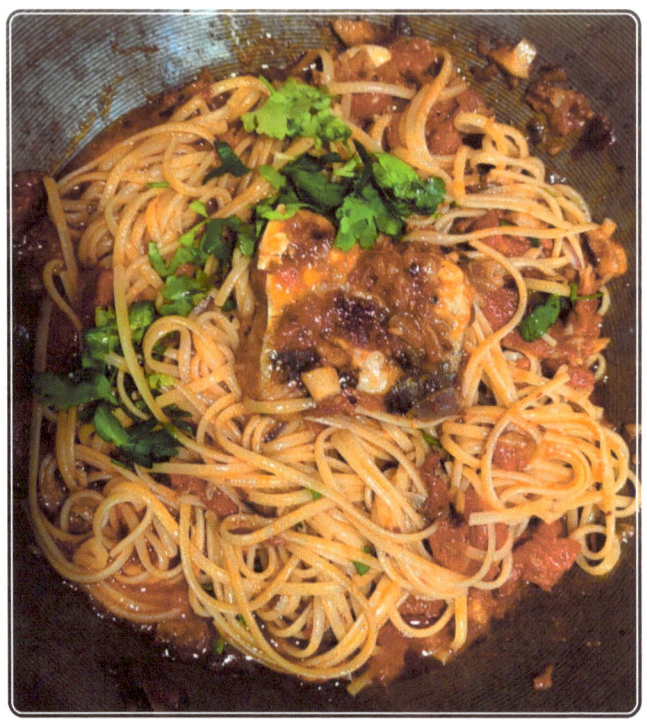

INGREDIENTS FOR 4 SERVINGS

1. 300 gr of quality salt cod fish in fillet already soaked.
2. 7/8 dry sweet red peppers.
3. 2 Tablespoons of quality tomato paste.
4. A sprig of parsley.
5. 5/6 tablespoons of olive oil.
6. 300 gr of quality "Linguine" pasta, not too narrow.
7. 2/3 tablespoons stale bread loaf crumb.
8. 1 organic lime.
9. A tuft of finely chopped parsley.
10. A pinch of freshly ground pepper.

DIRECTIONS

In a pan large enough to serve the linguine, heat the oil, sauté the garlic, and toast the sweet dried red peppers.

Prevent the oil from frying and burning the peppers.

Place the toasted peppers in the freezer for 7/8 minutes and then in a mortar, pestle them by adding a few tablespoons of oil where the peppers have been toasted, until a creamy mixture is obtained.

Cut the cod fillets into pieces and brown them in the oil of the pan. Deglaze the cod with a splash of white wine, better if a Brut Prosecco.

Add the creamy mixture of toasted peppers referred to in point 2. In a non-stick pan, toast the stale bread crumb until brown.

Cook the linguine in lightly salted water and pan fry "al dente" in the saucepan, adding, if necessary, some pasta cooking water.

Sprinkle the pasta with freshly ground pepper and toasted crumb. Grate a little lime peel on the crumb.

Add the chopped parsley and serve.

NOTE

Pay attention to the salting of the sauce and pasta, adjusting it according to the flavor of the salt cod fillets.

41) Spaghetti with sea urchins

INGREDIENTS

1. 12 Sea urchins per person.
2. Garlic, possibly fresh.
3. Chily in moderation.
4. Extra-virgin olive oil.
5. 80/100 Gr of quality spaghetti.
6. An organic lemon zest.
7. Chopped parsley.

DIRECTIONS

Open the sea urchins and with a teaspoon take the pulp and liquid and put them in a cup, or glass.

In a frying pan brown in oil a clove of garlic, chili pepper, a strip of lemon zest and a whole stalk of parsley.

Remove the ingredients when brown.

In the same browning oil, add a large amount of parsley.

Cook the spaghetti and stir-fry it in the, adding some spoonsful of pasta water.

Remove the pan from the heat, add the raw sea urchins to the spaghetti and grate a little lemon zest on top.

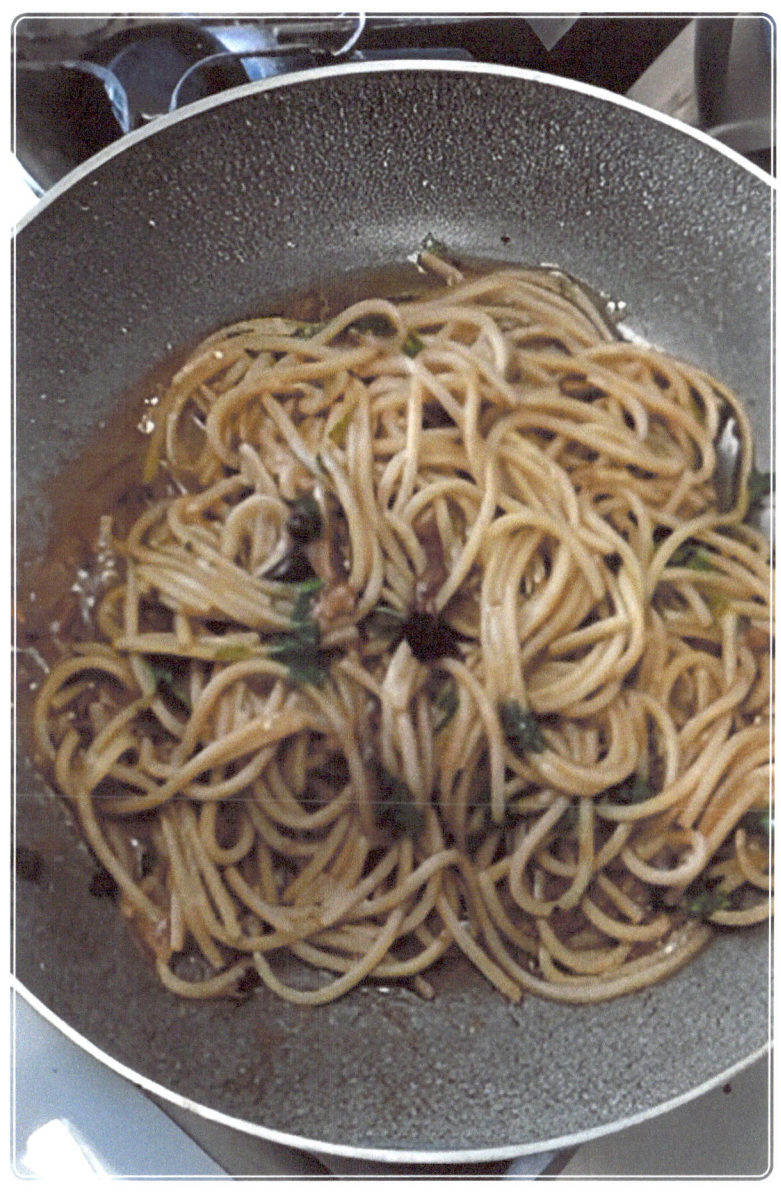

42) Stuffed sepia cuttlefish with caramelized onions

INGREDIENTS

1. One cuttlefish from the Adriatic per person.
2. One red onion of Tropea, every other cuttlefish.
3. One/two cloves of garlic.
4. Breadcrumb to fill cuttlefish. Extra virgin olive oil, and parsley.
5. One egg
6. 30grof good pecorino cheese.
7. Salt and pepper

PROCEDURE

Prepare the filling by mixing the wet and squeezed crumb, the beaten egg, the chopped garlic and parsley, some grated pecorino cheese, oil, salt, and pepper.

Fill the cuttlefish with the compound, which must be compact, and close them with toothpicks.

In a patch, fry the onions in sufficient oil over very low heat.

Put the cuttlefish on the fried onions and let them simmer in the water they will release.

Prolong cooking over very low heat, until the onions and cuttlefish are caramelized.

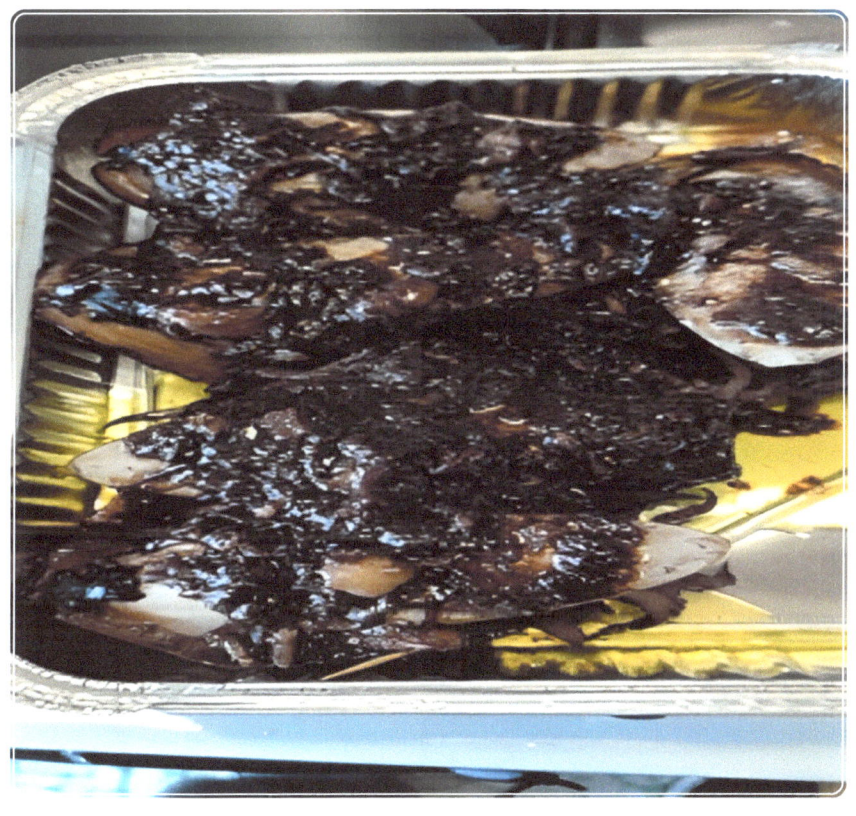

43) Marinated sepia and Scialatielli Pasta with sepia tentacles.

INGREDIENTS

1. One cuttlefish per person for large portions, otherwise only one is enough, for two people.
2. 4/5 dried sweet red peppers.
3. Some chopped parsley.
4. Half red onion.
5. 2/3 Spoonful of olive oil.
6. One Chili pepper.
7. A couple of tablespoons of good tomato paste.
8. A cup of hot water.

DIRECTIONS

Spread the cuttlefish on a cutting board and with a sharp filleting knife cut it horizontally to obtain thin and uniform layers.

Let the sepia soak in quality oil and then season it with Tropea red onion, fresh green chili pepper and a spray of good apple cider vinegar.

Serve the raw cuttlefish on slices of toasted bread.

Pasta sauce.
After roasting three dried sweet peppers per person in a little hot oil, when they cool, beat them in a mortar adding the roasting oil and some coarse salt grain, until you get a creamy mixture.

In a pan brown with garlic and parsley the tentacles of the cuttlefish (eight short tentacles and two long ones for each sepia).

Add to the browned sepia tentacles a tablespoon of good tomato paste, the creamy mixture of red dried peppers and one or two small cups of hot water.

Cook the Scialatielli Pasta and as soon as they are "al dente", drain and pour hem into the pan with the sauce.

Add some pasta cooking water if pasta is too dry.

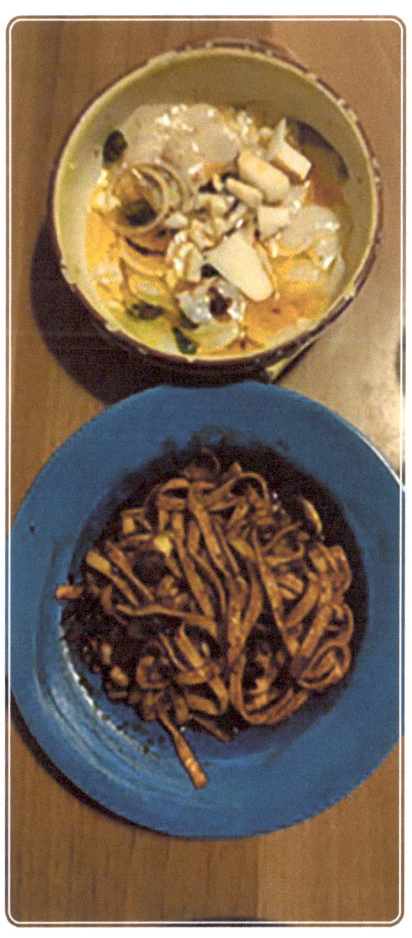

44) Pappardelle Pasta 3.0 with porcini mushrooms

INGREDIENTS FOR FOUR PEOPLE

1. 150 gr of veal, 150 gr of pork neck meat, 150 gr of lamb.
2. 15/20 gr of dry quality porcini mushrooms to soak in water. In the case of fresh porcini two three per person, if small, less, if large.
3. Ingredients for a vegetable broth, celery, onion, and more vegetables.
4. A little white dry wine next to.
5. Some grated Parmesan cheese.
6. Salt and pepper

DIRECTIONS

Cut the three pieces of different meat into small pieces.

Prepare one liter of vegetable broth.

Keep the porcini mushrooms one hour in water with a pinch of salt, until they become soft.

In a pan that can contain Pappardelle Pasta, make a light sauté with garlic, onion, parsley, and any aromatic herbs.

Sauté the minced meat.
Blend with little white wine.

Add the porcini mushrooms softened in the water.

Add a little salt and pepper in the sauce.

Cook the meat and mushrooms by adding some vegetable broth.

Cook the pappardelle for a few minutes in the vegetable broth.

Drain them and finish cooking by stirring them in the sauce, adding the vegetable stock in small quantities.

Serve with grated Parmesan Cheese and parsley.

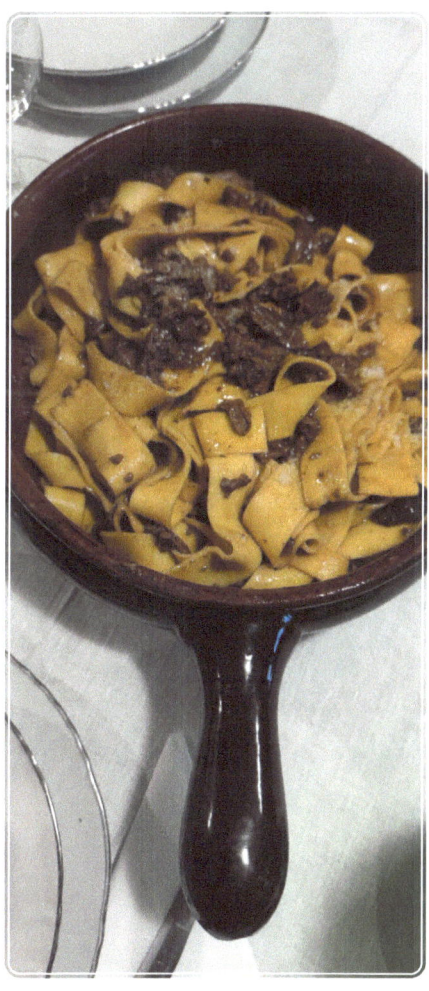

45) 3.0 Sauce for Pasta alla Mugnaia (The Miller's recipe)

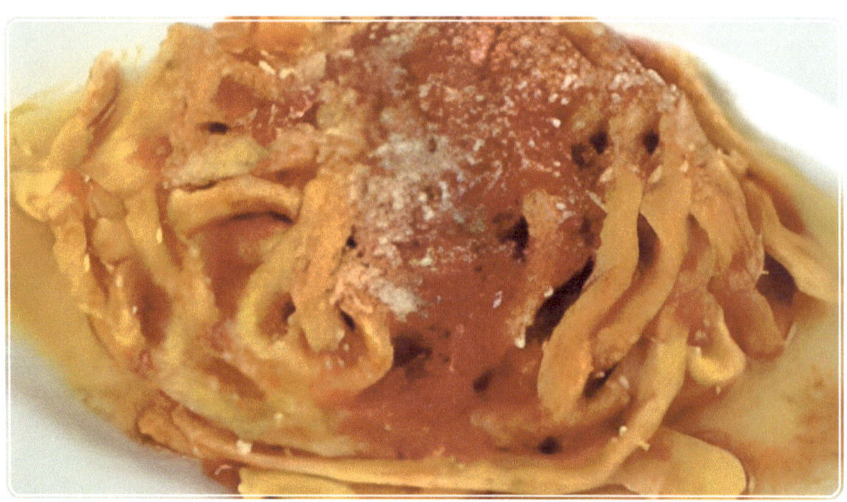

INGREDIENTS FOR FOUR PEOPLE

1. Pasta alla Mugnaia Kg 1 (Home made pasta
2. 150 gr of veal pulp, 150 gr of pork neck, 150 gr of lamb.
3. One/ two ox knee bones.
4. Ingredients, garlic, onion and any aromatic herb you like more to your.
5. Half a glass of white dry wine.
6. Tomato sauce 1.5 lt,
7. A tablespoon of tomato paste.
8. Salt and pepper
9. Grated Parmesan cheese

DIRECTIONS

In a pan make a light sauté with garlic, onion, and any herbs you like. Brown the three types of meat and bones.

Add half a glass of white dry wine and let it evaporate. Add and melt the half tablespoon of tomato paste in the fried mixture.

Add and cover with the tomato sauce the meat and the bones. Add salt and pepper to your taste.

Cook everything over very slow heat, until a thick sauce is obtained. Cook the pasta and season it first with Parmesan, then with the sauce and finally with some more grated Parmesan.

46) Maltagliati Pasta with Garbanzo beans, clams, mussels, and cuttlefish

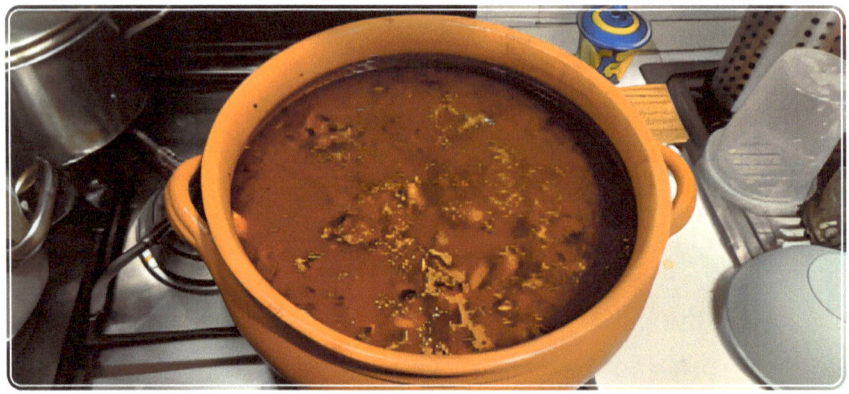

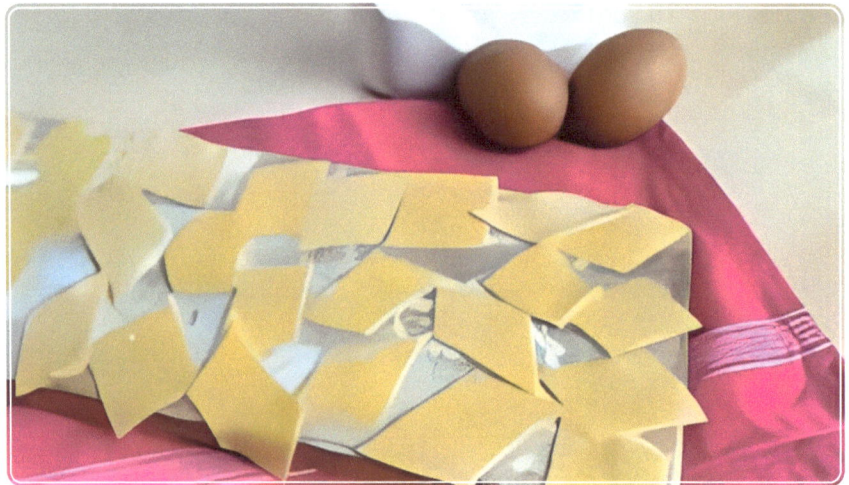

INGREDIENTS FOR FOUR PEOPLE

1. 500 gr. of Maltagliati, or Tacconelli home made pasta
2. 4/5 Red dried sweet peppers.
3. 250grof Garbanzo beans.
4. A peeled garlic.
5. 2/3 tablespoons of tomato paste.

6. One kg of mussels
7. ½ kg of Adriatic clams.
8. A strip of fresh green pepper
9. Extra virgin olive oil.

DIRECTIONS OF THE DISHOF THE DISH

In a pan pour a spoonful of olive oil per person and the peeled garlic. Heat the oil and toast the dried red peppers, one each two people. (See Toasting the Fuffulloni in the recipe book.)

Grind in a mortar the toasted dried red peppers, the garlic and some oil used for toasting. In another pan open the clams and the mussels.

When cool shell them and filter the water. Keep the Garbanzo beans in water for one night, in water. Boil them in water with laurel, garlic dress and little salt, until they soften slightly.

In the oil used to toast the red dry peppers brown the cuttlefish cut into small pieces, one for each person. Add the tablespoons of tomato paste and mix. Add the Garbanzo beans in a little cooking water.

Add the shelled mussels, the clams, and their filtered water. Mix everything together for a few minutes.

Cook the Scialatielli pasta "al dente" drain it and pour into the sauce, which will be brothy, but thick.

Attention to salt, due to the sapidity of the fruit waters, only half tea spoonful of salt will be enough to salt the water for cooking pasta.

47) Tubetti or short pasta, potatoes, and seafood.

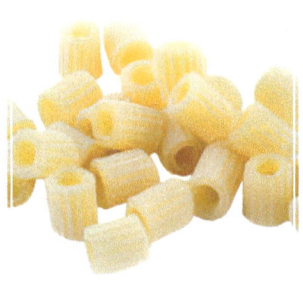 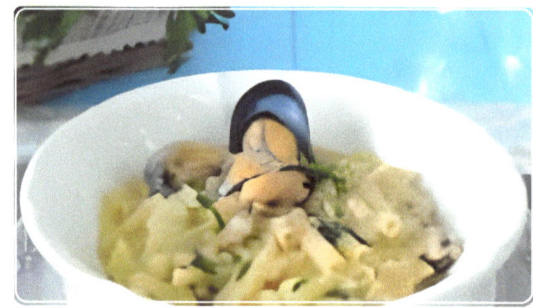

INGREDIENTS FOR FOUR PEOPLE

1. 1 potato per person
2. 500 gr mussels
3. 500 gr of clams from the Adriatic sea (if not available common clams will do)
4. 300 gr Tubetti, or other short pasta
5. Extra virgin olive oil
6. Garlic and parsley
7. Two, three strips of green pepper.
8. 1/2 glass of dry white wine
9. A sprig of rosemary
10. Salt, pepper, and hot green pepper if it is season.

DIRECTIONS OF THE DISH

In a pan put a drizzle of oil, a clove of garlic and the sprig of rosemary.

When the garlic browns, add the fruits, blend with a little white wine, and then add a half glass of water.

When the fruits open, remove them from the fire and peel them. Continue to boil the water of the fruits making it withdraw a little.

Veil the bottom of a pan with a drizzle of oil. Brown two, three cloves of garlic cut into slices. Put the potatoes cut into slices of half a cm a pinch of salt. Sauté the potatoes for a few minutes adding the cooking liquid of the fruits.

Cover the potatoes with hot water and cook them until they soften.

Cook the Tubetti "al dente" drain and put the Pasta in the pan with the potatoes.

Add the shelled sea fruits.

Sprinkle with parsley the pasta.

Let it cool before serving.

48) Bucatini alla trescatora

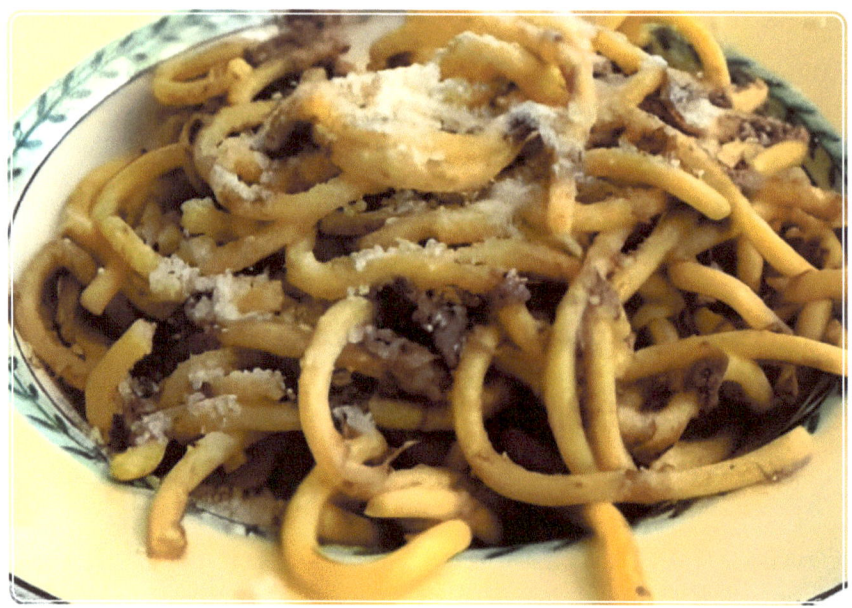

INGREDIENTS

1. Half duck with guts; heart and liver (if you like).
2. Extra virgin olive oil, pepper, and salt.
3. Aromatic herbs; rosemary, thyme, marjoram, half white onion, and garlic.
4. 1 kg of tomato sauce, or a bottle of homemade tomato.
5. A spoonful of quality tomato paste.
6. Grated quality Pecorino from Abruzzo.
7. 80 gr of Bucatini per person.

Flavor the duck with the above ingredients, as 1 and 2.

Spread it on oven paper and bake at 200°for about an hour until it is well browned.

While cooking the duck, in a pan fry the guts in oil and garlic. When the duck is cooked cut it into pieces.

Choose the least fleshy pieces: wings, neck, and feet and put them in a pan.
Add a tablespoon of quality tomato paste and mix with the pieces.
Add the fried guts and stir the mixture.

Cover all the sautéed pieces with fresh tomato sauce.
Bring the sauce to a boil.

Reduce the flame and let sauce cook for two or more hours.
The sauce will be ready as soon as the olive oil starts boiling and comes up to the surface of the sauce.

Season the bucatini "al dente" the with the sauce and add the pecorino cheese.
Serve as second dish the duck and its guts with fried potatoes.

49) Spaghetti according to the Miller's recipe offered during the milling.

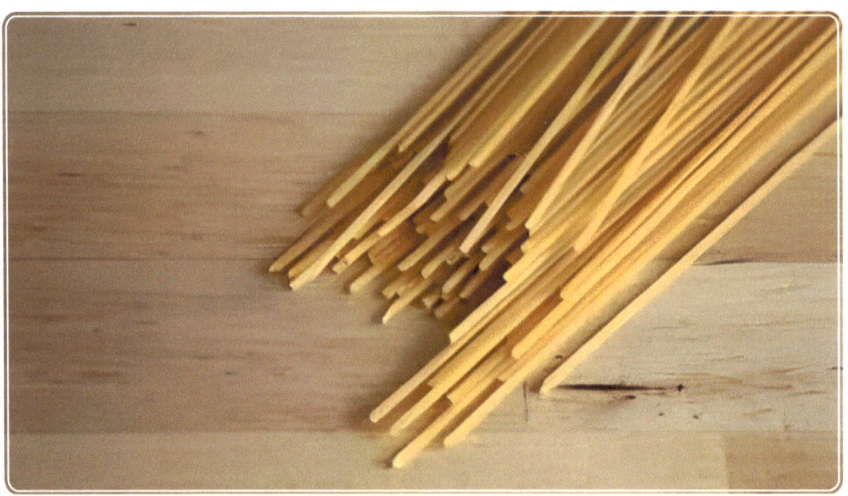

INGREDIENTS

1. 2 spoonsful Extra Virgin Olive Oil, from the new milling.
2. 2 cloves of peeled garlic per person.
3. 2 Salted Anchovies, or sardines per person.
4. 1 Spoonful of ground crumbled bread per person.
5. 3 Green fresh olives per person.
6. Half a tablespoon of sweet dried red peppers per person.
7. Some chopped parsley and mint.
8. Red hot dried pepper

DIRECTIONS

In a frying pan brown the peeled cloves of garlic in olive oil.

Add the anchovies, or sardines and melt them.

Add the fresh olives pitted.

Add the chopped sweet and dry pepper.

In a non-stick pan toast the bread crumb.

Cook the spaghetti "al dente" and season with the sauce.

Serve the pasta with the toasted crumb, and on top.

50) Spaghetti, or Linguine with tuna in oil

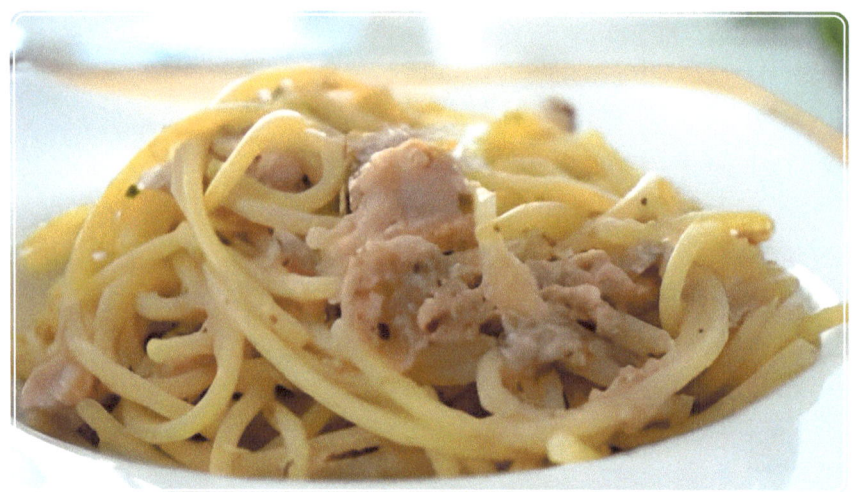

INGREDIENTS

1. 2 Spoonsful of Extra-virgin olive oil per person.
2. 1/2 peeled clove of garlic.
3. 2/ 3 Spoonsful of chopped parsley.
4. 2 Spoonsful of chopped salted capers desalted in water.
5. 1 Piccadilly cherry tomato, or Pachino per person.
6. 1 Spoonful of oregano, better if fresh.
7. 3/4 Pitted olive per person.
8. 2 Cans of quality tuna fish in olive oil.
9. 3/4 Spoonsful of grated and toasted breadcrumbs.

DIRECTIONS

In a frying pan, add garlic and parsley.

Remove them, if you do not like, when browned.

Add the capers, chopped cherry tomatoes and pitted olives.

Cook the mixture over low heat at the same time as cooking the pasta.

Drain the pasta "al dente".

Finish the cooking by sautéing it in the mixture, if necessary, add some cooking water.

Out of the heat, add the tuna in oil and sprinkle the dish with oregano and chopped parsley.

51) Paella revisited

INGREDIENTS for 3/4 people of normal appetite

1. 500 gr of Carnaroli rice
2. 4/5 Small green peppers.
3. 5/6 Cloves of d garlic
4. 1 Shallot
5. A couple of tablespoons of sweet paprika, or Spanish paprika powder.
6. A spoonful of quality tomato paste.
7. A liter and a half of vegetable and fish broth; made boiling in salted water for twenty minute some chopped celery, parsley, carrot, scampi heads, some mussel and some clams.
8. A few stalks parsley.
9. Half a sprig of rosemary.
10. Half a glass of white wine
11. A handful of peas and some green beans if you like.
12. A small bag of saffron.
13. 1 Spoonful Olive oil per person.
14. A little salt and pepper.
15. A pork neck steak.
16. 3/4 Small pieces of rabbit.
17. 3/4 Small pieces of chicken breast.
18. Half a kg of mussels
19. A handful of clams
20. 8/10 Scampi
21. 8/10 Squillas (Cicala di mare).
22. A medium-sized cuttlefish (Sepia).

DIRECTIONS

In large iron pan, in oil enough, brown the cloves of garlic and a chopped shallot and fry the
Red small peppers cut into pieces.

Following the order, first squeeze the head of the scampi into the fried base and set it aside after it has been well squeezed.

Fry one after the other all the ingredients as listed above 15,16,17.

Add the paprika in small quantities.

Stir the spoonsful of tomato paste in the fry. The sauté must be pink and not red.

In another pan, in a drizzle of olive oil brown a little parsley, a couple garlic cloves and a half sprig of rosemary fry part of the mussels and clams, the scampi, and a cup of water.

Leave aside some not shelled mussels and clams to serve on top.

As soon as the mussels and clams open, remove them from the fire.

Open the mussels and clams.

Set aside the cooking water after filtering, if necessary. This water is valuable for giving rice its first wetting.

Prepare a vegetable broth by adding to the usual ingredients of the vegetable broth the heads of the scampi squeezed with all the claws, the mussels and clams left aside, and a pinch of salt.

Let the broth reduce until it becomes tasty.

In the fried food made previously, toast the rice, after washing it. When toasted, water it with the water of the mussels and the clams.

When the water dries proceed with cooking the rice by covering it with broth.
Repeat the wetting until the rice is cooked.

Add the saffron melted in hot water.

Add some mussels and clams with the shell to the rice, prawns, chops, mussels, and clams.
Wait for a slight cooling of the rice, for when hot does not allow you to taste the amalgam of the flavors.

Serve the rice accompanied by a mousse of garlic and oil passed to the pimer.

52) Sea bass in salt crust

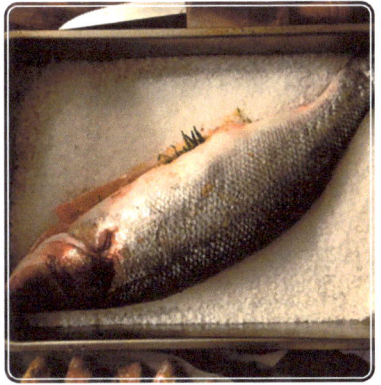 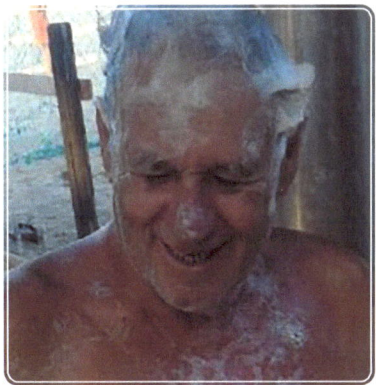

Cooked in this way just to please a friend.

INGREDIENTS FOR 4 people

1. One 1 Kg Sea bass
2. Two Kg of coarse salt
3. 400 g of egg white
4. One Lemmon zest
5. One Orange zest
6. A bunch of rosemary
7. Eight gr White pepper
8. Four gr of fenkel powder, or a small bunch of leaves
9. Four Spoonsful of Extra Virgin Olive oil
10. Four Spoonsful of chopped parsley
11. One and a half spoonful of salted capers
12. Three/four anchovies in oil
13. Two spoonsful of breadcrumb
14. Two spoonsful of white wine vinegar.
15. Two ice cubes
16. Two peeled cloves of garlic

Start beating the egg whites with a mixer.
Put the egg whites in a bowl add the coarse salt, the herbs and mix.

Remove the guts from the sea bass.
Put on an oven pan a part of the mixed salt sale, lay on it the sea bass and cover it with the remaining part of the salt.

Make three, four cuts under the sea bass gills.
Fill them with the cloves of garlic and some chopped parsley.
Cook in the oven at 170° for 25 minutes.

Nel frattempo, preparare la salsa verde mettendo nel mixer prezzemolo capperi mollica ammollata nell'aceto, cubetti di ghiaccio e olio extravergine. Frullare e servire come salsa per condire la spigola.

Meanwhile, blend with an electric mixer the parsley, the capers, the breadcrumb soaked in water. Serve the sauce on top of the sea bass.

www.ingramcontent.com/pod-product-compliance
Lightning Source LLC
Chambersburg PA
CBHW040846120626

46547CB00001B/45